HEALTHY SOUP RECIPES

HEALTHY SOUP RECIPES

QUICK, EASY AND DELICIOUS RECIPES
FOR HEALTHY SOUPS

JAGO HOLMES CPT

HEALTHY SOUP RECIPES

QUICK, EASY AND DELICIOUS RECIPES FOR HEALTHY SOUPS

by Jago Holmes CPT

Copyright @ 2023 New Image Fitness Ltd

Book design by Vesna Mitic

Available on www.amazon.com

CONTENTS

BEEF SOUP RECIPES

PORK SOUP RECIPE

CHICKEN SOUP RECIPES

SEAFOOD SOUP RECIPES

FISH SOUP RECIPES

VEGETARIAN SOUP RECIPES

VEGAN SOUP RECIPES

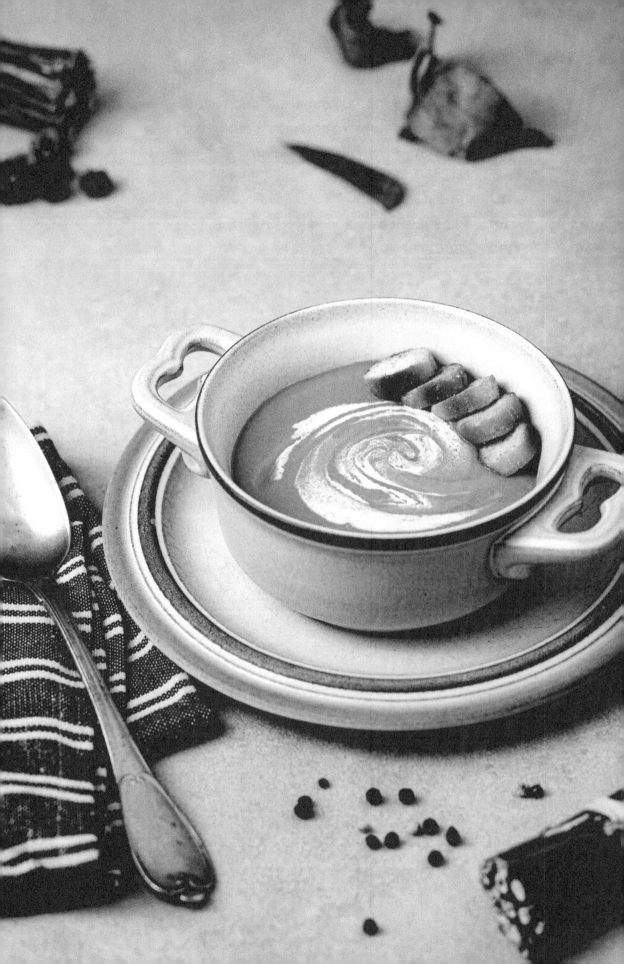

HELLO, MY NAME IS **JAGO HOLMES**

I'm a personal trainer and weight loss expert here at New Image Fitness Ltd in the UK.

I'd like to offer you a very warm welcome to my new book, '*Soup Recipes -Quick, Easy And Delicious Recipes For Healthy Soups.*' In this comprehensive recipe book, I've featured a wide range of soups that are not only delicious, but also easy to prepare. The recipes have been carefully selected to be healthy and satisfying -without the need for too many added fats or sugars.

Whilst the vast majority of the soups in this book are very healthy, I've included some recipes that may not be considered low in fat. As with all diets, enjoying foods that are higher in sugar or fat every so often won't harm you -as long as most of what you eat is a well-balanced mixture of nutritious foods which are naturally low in fat, salt, and sugar.

Soups are an excellent choice for those who care about their health and fitness because they can offer a wealth of vitamins and minerals without the preservatives, sugars, and fats typically found in most processed or convenience foods.

You'll find that these recipes are extremely quick and easy to prepare, with most having relatively short cooking times.

It's quite difficult to go wrong with a soup, especially when you have a recipe to follow, and getting organized by preparing all the ingredients before you start cooking simplifies the process even further.

Another significant advantage of soups is that they are very cost-effective compared to typical meals. They're also highly versatile and can often be adapted slightly, by changing the ingredients without making a noticeable difference to the overall taste.

The only equipment you'll need is a food processor or a hand-held blender. I prefer the hand-held version because it's less cumbersome and you don't have to transfer the soup to a processor; you can blend it right in the pan. Plus, it saves on washing up!

You'll notice that some of these recipes contain a thickening agent such as potatoes, which when added will provide the starch needed to thicken them. If you'd rather not use potatoes, you can use cornflour or plain flour instead, mixed with a little water, added gradually to the soup while stirring continuously.

Also, if you want to reduce the fat content in soups containing milk or cream, it's an easy fix! Simply replace the milk or cream with extra vegetable, beef, chicken, or fish stock instead.

Top Tip: When preparing a soup, make a larger batch and freeze what you're not going to use the same day. This way, you'll have a supply of nutritious, healthy meals you can control, knowing exactly what's in them. It's a quick option; just take it out of the freezer the evening before. This will help prevent you from resorting to takeaways or ready-made meals as a quick fix when you can't be bothered to cook yourself.

I hope you thoroughly enjoy making and eating these soups as much as I have enjoyed creating, testing, and writing them myself.

CHAPTER 1

EXPLORING THE WORLD OF SOUPS

In the realm of gastronomy, few dishes possess the simplicity and versatility of soups. They are the culinary blank canvas upon which flavors are painted and provide the cozy warmth of taste and textures that soothe the soul on a cold winter's day.

As we embark on this journey through a rich tapestry of soups, you will discover the many layers of taste, different cultures, and nourishment that define this humble yet exciting and highly accessible dish.

The Genesis of Soup

The history of soup is as ancient as human civilization itself. The word "soup" is derived from the old French word "soupe," which means "bread soaked in broth." It's a humble beginning, born of necessity when resourceful cooks discovered that simmering ingredients in a communal pot could transform even the most meager of provisions into a nourishing and tasty meal. From this modest start, the world of soups has evolved over the centuries into an art form encompassing a kaleidoscope of flavors, textures, and traditions.

Throughout this book, we will delve deeper into the world of soups, traversing continents, and cultures, each contributing its unique chapter to the story. From the aromatic Pho of Vietnam to the hearty Minestrone of Italy, the fiery Tom Yum of Thailand to the comforting chicken noodle of America, soups offer a passport to travel through the world of great taste.

The Magic of Broth

At the heart of every soup lies its liquid foundation, the broth or stock. Whether it's a clear consommé, a creamy bisque, or a robust stew, the choice of broth is a critical decision in crafting the perfect soup. It can be a simple chicken stock, a complex bone marrow elixir, or a flavorful vegetable brew, but its role is undeniable. The broth holds the power to transform ordinary ingredients into a symphony of flavors, infusing warmth, and comfort into every mouthful.

From the Garden to the Bowl

Soups can be created from a bountiful garden of ingredients. Fresh vegetables, fragrant herbs, tender meats, and exotic spices all have their place in the soup pot. As we explore various recipes, we'll witness how these elements combine to create harmonious flavor profiles, providing sustenance and satisfaction in every mouth full.

Soup-making is a process that balances relatively simple cooking techniques with intuition. Whether you're following a cherished family recipe passed down through generations or experimenting with newfound ingredients, the art of preparation lies at the heart of every soup. From the precise chopping of ingredients to the patient simmering on a stove, it's a mindful process that culminates in a dish that warms both body and spirit.

Beyond Sustenance: Soup as a Cultural Symbol

Beyond its culinary significance, soup often serves as a symbol of culture, community, and belonging. It's the dish that brings families together at the dinner table, the offering that extends hospitality to guests, and the remedy that offers solace during times of illness. Soup's symbolism is as rich as its taste.

In the chapters that follow, we'll uncover the secrets of crafting the perfect broth, explore diverse regional variations, and learn how to follow both classic and innovative soup recipes. Whether you're a seasoned chef or a novice cook, during our time together we will celebrate the long-held appeal of soups and the joy of sharing them with loved ones.

So, ladle in hand and apron donned, let's go to a place where nourishment meets artistry, where tradition meets innovation, and where every simmering pot holds the promise of an exciting new flavorful discovery.

CHAPTER 2

. . . .

TO BLEND OR NOT TO BLEND - THE SECRET CODE OF SOUPS

In the world of food, few dishes exhibit the artistry of flavors, textures, and aromas quite like soups. These liquid canvases, enriched with an array of ingredients and seasonings, have the power to nourish not only our bodies but also our souls. Yet, there exists a subtle, often overlooked question -to blend or not to blend?

Picture this: A rustic, chunky minestrone, brimming with hearty vegetables and pasta, each spoonful delivering a unique blend of flavors and textures. Contrast it with a velvety butternut squash bisque; its silky consistency caressing your palate as the subtle sweetness of the squash dances with the warmth of spices. Both are soups, but each has a very different personality.

The decision to blend or maintain the integrity of individual ingredients is a culinary crossroads that defines the very character of a soup. It is a choice that hinges on texture, flavor, and the desired dining experience. Ultimately it is a personal choice, a decision of preference based on a certain mood, time of year, the ingredients available or the company the soup is to be eaten with. All may lead to the decision of how to present the soup at the table.

Blending is the process that transforms a medley of ingredients into a harmonious symphony of flavors. It unites vegetables, meats, legumes, herbs, and spices into a silky-smooth blend that bathes the palate in a consistent, well-balanced meal. Creamy soups, such as veloutés and purées, owe their velvety textures to this process. Here, ingredients are meticulously emulsified, resulting in a luxurious taste sensation that coats the tongue with every spoonful.

But blending is not solely about creating uniformity. It's also a tool that improves the infusion of flavors, blending ingredients into a union that transcends their individuality. It transforms humble vegetables into rich bisques and vibrant gazpachos, where the freshness of tomatoes and the bite of peppers merge into an unforgettable taste.

The Beauty of Texture

Yet, in the world of soups, texture is a treasure. The decision not to blend is an invitation for ingredients to express their unique qualities. Imagine a French onion soup with tender caramelized onions, topped with a crusty layer of melted cheese and bread, a sensory journey from the crispy top to the delicate threads below. Here, texture is as vital as the taste itself, and each bite offers a new revelation.

In broths and consommés, clarity reigns supreme. The refusal to blend allows ingredients to shine in their pristine form, where the transparency of the broth reflects the purity of flavors. From the delicate strands of egg in a classic Chinese egg drop soup to the intricate dance of herbs in a Vietnamese pho, these unblended concoctions are an ode to the unique essence and characteristics of the ingredients.

Ultimately the choice to blend or not to blend is yours alone – there is no right or wrong answer, only your mood or decision on that day will decide. So do whichever you like, and don't be afraid to experiment with different textures. Remember, it really is genuinely difficult to ruin a soup!

In the chapters that follow, we will explore recipes that celebrate both blended and unblended soups. From classic veloutés to hearty stews, from broths that soothe the soul to thick chowders that warm the heart, we will look at all methods and styles of soup-making.

CHAPTER 3

REPLACING INGREDIENTS IN SOUPS

Soup is a versatile and very forgiving dish, making it an excellent blank canvas for creativity in the kitchen. Whether you're accommodating dietary restrictions, using up leftovers, or experimenting with flavors, knowing how to replace ingredients in soups can lead to exciting and delicious results. In this chapter, we'll look more closely at ingredient replacements that can transform your soups while maintaining their core taste and flavor.

1. Broth or Stock Substitutes

Vegetable Broth: For a vegetarian or vegan twist, replace meat or fish-based broths and stocks with vegetable broth. It adds depth and flavor while aligning with plant-based diets.

Mushroom Broth: Introduce a rich, earthy character to your soups by using mushroom broth. It's an excellent choice for enhancing umami flavors.

Seafood Stock: Supercharge seafood soups by substituting seafood stock for chicken or vegetable broth. It imparts a delightful oceanic flavor.

There are basically a couple of options for each of the above:

1. Shop bought stock or broth: Either in the form of cubes, bouillon powder or fresh stock-found in the refrigerated section of your local supermarket, or

2. Homemade Stock or Broth: Crafting your own broth from kitchen scraps and vegetable peels, onion skins, and herb stems is both sustainable and flavorful. In the next chapter, we'll take a quick look at how to make a homemade broth for yourself. Not that you need to do it this way, as there are many great shop bought products, but if you'd like to give it a go, you can learn exactly how to do it there.

2. Protein Substitutes

If a recipe calls for meat or fish, but you want to make it using an alternative instead, that's fine. Here are a range of protein options you can choose from:

Tofu: Replace meat or poultry with tofu for a protein-packed, plant-based option. Press and dice firm tofu, then season and sauté it before adding (it) to your soup.

Lentils: Lentils are a fantastic source of plant-based protein. They work well in hearty soups and stews, adding texture and substance along with a real honesty and warmth of flavor.

Legumes: Beans, such as black beans, kidney beans, or chickpeas, are a great protein alternative. Canned or cooked beans can be easily incorporated into soups.

Seitan: Seitan, often referred to as *"wheat meat,"* is a protein-rich meat substitute that can be diced and added to soups for a meaty texture.

3. Cream or Dairy Replacements

There are many reasons why you might want to replace dairy with an alternative, such as to reduce the total calories, to avoid lactose for those with intolerances or on ethical grounds.

Whatever the decision to look for replacements, the good news is that there are plenty of them easily available these days. You can use any of the following:

Coconut Milk: For a dairy-free and creamy consistency, use coconut milk in place of heavy cream. It adds a delightful tropical flavor to certain soups.

Cashew Cream: Soaked and blended cashews create a creamy, dairy-free alternative. Add it at the end of cooking for a silky finish.

Greek Yogurt: Swap heavy cream or sour cream with fat-free Greek yogurt for a tangy, protein-rich option. Whilst this is still obviously dairy, it will substantially reduce the calorie content of the soup when compared to using cream instead. Removing the soup from the heat before stirring in the yogurt will prevent curdling.

4. Vegetable Alternatives

This is an easy one. If you see a recipe that you like the look of, but you're out of a key vegetable ingredient, don't sweat it, just switch out the one you've got instead. Here are some options for you:

Leafy Greens: Swap spinach or kale for more traditional greens like collard greens, cabbage, or Swiss chard. Leafy greens add color, nutrients, and a pleasant slight bitterness to soups.

Sweet Potatoes: Replace regular potatoes with sweet potatoes for a sweeter, nutrient-dense twist. They work well in both creamy and broth-based soups.

Zoodles: Spiralized zucchini, known as 'zoodles', can replace pasta in soups, offering a lighter, low-carb alternative.

5. Seasoning Substitutes

We'll cover this in a little more detail later on, but here are a few alternatives you can use if you run out of key seasoning ingredients:

Dried Herbs: When fresh herbs are unavailable, dried herbs can be used instead. Remember that dried herbs are more potent, so use them sparingly.

Spice Blends: If a particular spice blend is missing from your pantry, mix your own using individual spices. Experiment with ratios until you achieve the desired flavor.

Citrus Zest: Freshly grated/finely shredded citrus zest is a good option as it imparts a wonderfully concentrated burst of citrus flavor into your soup.

6. Allergen-Friendly Swaps

If you or someone you're cooking soups for has intolerances or allergies, then here are a few swaps you can try:

Gluten-Free Pasta: Replace traditional pasta with gluten-free varieties like rice noodles, quinoa pasta, or chickpea pasta to accommodate gluten sensitivities.

Nut-Free Alternatives: If a recipe calls for nuts, consider sunflower seeds, pumpkin seeds, or roasted chickpeas instead for adding texture and crunch.

Dairy Yogurt: There are lots of replacements to these available, some of the best are coconut or oat-based yogurts.

7. Turn Leftovers Into a Hearty Lunch

Instead of throwing away leftovers from a family meal, why not use them in a soup the next day? You're almost guaranteed to find a recipe in this book that you can add yesterday's leftovers to.

Use Leftover Protein: Utilize cooked chicken, turkey, or beef from previous meals to create flavorful and hearty soups.

Repurpose Vegetables: Leftover roasted or steamed vegetables can be added to soups for extra nutrients and flavor.

In the world of soup-making, there are endless possibilities for ingredient substitutions and very rarely are there any definite 'right' and 'wrongs.' You can get creative and adapt recipes to your preferences and dietary needs. Keep experimenting, and you'll discover unique and delicious flavor combinations that will keep your soup repertoire exciting and satisfying.

CHAPTER 4

· ·

HOW TO MAKE HOMEMADE BROTHS

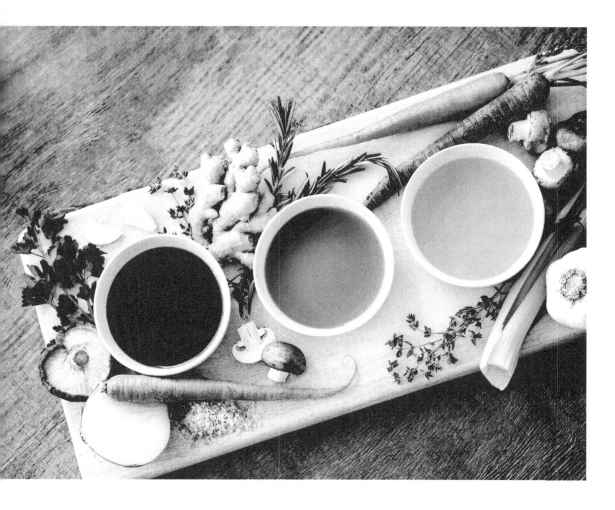

Homemade broth or stock is the secret ingredient that can elevate your soups to the next level. It's the foundation of countless dishes, from soups and stews to risottos and sauces. Creating your own broth or stock from scratch isn't difficult to do and it allows you to control the flavors, quality, and nutritional content, while reducing food waste by using leftover ingredients. In this chapter, we'll take you through the simple steps of crafting this essential kitchen staple. For our example we'll use a protein-based stock. This could be chicken, beef, pork, seafood, or fish.

Ingredients:

Bones and Scraps: To make a protein-based broth or stock, you'll need bones and scraps from poultry, beef, pork, or fish. These can be raw or cooked, and you can mix and match for a more complex flavor.

Vegetables: Onions, carrots, and celery are the classic choices. But you can also add garlic, leeks, mushrooms, and herbs like parsley, thyme, and bay leaves for a deeper depth of flavor.

Water: Good quality water is crucial for achieving a clean, pure taste.

Equipment:

Stockpot or Large Pot: Use a pot large enough to accommodate your ingredients comfortably.

Strainer or Cheesecloth: You'll need a way to strain the solids from your finished broth or stock.

Storage Containers: Have a few airtight containers or jars on hand for storing your homemade broth or stock when it has cooled. Freeze your soup in an airtight plastic container – a rectangular or square shape is easier to stack in the freezer.

Method:

Gather Your Ingredients: Collect your bones and vegetable scraps before you start, you'll need a good half pot full. If you're using raw bones, consider roasting them in the oven first at 400°F (200°C) for about 30 minutes until they turn golden brown as this step enhances the depth of flavor.

Combine Ingredients in the Pot: Place your bones and scraps in the stockpot. Add your vegetables and herbs. You can be generous with your additions; they'll impart their own flavors to the broth.

Cover with Water: Pour cold water over the ingredients until they are fully submerged. The water-to-ingredients ratio can vary, but a good rule of thumb is about 2 quarts (2 liters) of water for every 1 pound (450 grams) of bones.

Simmer Gently: Place the pot over a low heat and bring the mixture to a simmer. As soon as it begins to simmer, reduce the heat to maintain a gentle, steady simmer. Do not let it boil vigorously, as this can make the broth cloudy.

Skim off Impurities: As your broth simmers, foam and impurities may rise to the surface. Skim these off with a slotted spoon or fine mesh skimmer to keep your broth clear.

Simmer and Reduce: Let your broth simmer for several hours to extract maximum flavor. Chicken or poultry broth may take 2-3 hours, while beef or pork broth might simmer for 4-6 hours. Fish broth, being more delicate, can be ready in 1-2 hours, so be patient!

Strain Your Broth: Once your broth has simmered to your satisfaction, carefully strain it through a fine-mesh strainer or cheesecloth into another pot or large bowl. Discard any solids.

Cool and Store: Allow the soup to cool to room temperature, then refrigerate. As it cools, any excess fat will rise to the surface and solidify, making it easy to remove. Store the cooled broth in airtight containers in the refrigerator for up to a week or freeze it for several months.

Homemade broth or stock is a versatile kitchen staple that adds depth and richness to a wide range of dishes. By following these simple steps and customizing your ingredients, you can create a flavorful base for all of your soups while minimizing food waste and enjoying the satisfaction of homemade goodness in your cooking.

CHAPTER 5

. . . .

CREAMY SOUP SHORTCUTS:
ADDING TASTE WITHOUT THE CALORIES

Creamy soups have a way of comforting the soul. Their velvety texture and rich flavors can make a simple meal feel like a luxurious experience. Traditionally, cream and butter have been the go-to ingredients for achieving that luscious creaminess, but what if you're looking for healthier or dairy-free alternatives?

In this chapter, we'll explore a variety of replacement ingredients and techniques to make your soups taste irresistibly creamy while accommodating different dietary needs.

1. Coconut Milk: The Dairy-Free Delight

One of the most popular dairy alternatives for cream laden soups is coconut milk. It brings a subtle, tropical flavor that pairs well with many ingredients and is also much lower in calories and saturated fat than dairy cream. When using coconut milk, opt for the full-fat variety for the creamiest results or low fat to keep it healthy and lower cal. A good trick is to refrigerate the can and then skim off the thick coconut cream that rises to the top. This can be used to create an extra-rich soup texture, similar to double cream.

2. Cashew Cream: The Nutty Elixir

Cashew cream is another fantastic dairy substitute. Simply soak raw cashews for a few hours or overnight, then blend them with water until smooth. This cashew cream can be added to your soup to create a silky, creamy consistency. It's an excellent choice for those who prefer a neutral flavor that won't overpower the other ingredients.

3. Silken Tofu: The Protein Powerhouse

Silken tofu is an incredible thickening agent that also adds a protein boost to your soup. Blend it into your soup base until it's smooth and creamy. Silken tofu has a neutral taste, making it perfectly adaptable to various soup flavors. It's an excellent choice for vegan and vegetarian recipes.

4. Greek Yogurt: The Tangy Twist

If you're not strictly following a dairy-free diet, Greek yogurt can be a fantastic addition to creamy soups. It brings a delightful tanginess that complements savory flavors. Stir in Greek yogurt just before serving to maintain its creamy texture and prevent curdling. It's a protein-packed choice that works well in both hot and cold soups and the fat-free version is just as thick and creamy, only without the extra calories.

5. Nutritional Yeast: The Cheesy Alternative

Derived from Saccharomyces cerevisiae, a yeast variety cultivated on molasses, nutritional yeast undergoes a meticulous process. After cultivation, it is carefully harvested, washed, and dried with heat, a vital step that deactivates it. This deactivation is essential as it transforms nutritional yeast into a non-leavening agent, making it unsuitable for causing bread or other baked goods to rise.

In the realm of dairy-free cuisine, nutritional yeast emerges as the ultimate secret weapon for imparting a rich, cheesy essence to your dishes. Particularly valued in vegan cooking, as it closely replicates the nuanced flavor of cheese. When incorporating into your creamy soups, simply sprinkle a bit while blending, and marvel at the profound depth of taste it effortlessly introduces. Your soups will be transformed into delectable, plant-based masterpieces, thanks to this ingenious ingredient.

6. Potato Magic: Natural Creaminess

Potatoes have an incredible ability to lend natural creaminess to soups. Dice and boil a starchy potato until it's soft, then blend it into your soup. This method not only thickens your soup but also adds a subtle, earthy sweetness. It's a trick used in classic potato and leek soup, among others.

7. Roux: The Classic Thickener

A roux is a traditional French thickening agent made from equal parts flour and fat, usually butter. For a dairy-free version, substitute a plant-based fat like olive oil or coconut oil. Simply cook the fat and flour together in a small pan until they form a paste. Cook for 2 minutes and remove from the heat. Add a tablespoon of your soup to the roux and whisk till smooth, then whisk this mixture into your soup. It not only thickens the soup, but also imparts a delightful richness.

8. Corn-starch: Quick and Easy

If you're looking for a gluten-free thickening agent, corn-starch is your answer. Create a paste by mixing corn-starch with a small amount of cold liquid (like water or broth) and then whisk into your soup. Be sure to gently heat your soup after adding the corn-starch to activate its thickening power.

9. Blending Tricks: The Smooth Finish

Whether you're using dairy or dairy-free ingredients, a high-powered blender can be your best friend for achieving a silky-smooth and creamy texture. Blend your soup in batches and be cautious with hot liquids to avoid getting splashed.

10. The Finish Line: Simmer and Season

Once you've incorporated your creamy element, allow your soup to simmer gently to blend the flavors together thoroughly and thicken further if needed. Don't forget to season generously with salt and pepper to taste and add any herbs or spices that complement your soup's ingredients.

Remember that the key to a perfect creamy soup is balance. Experiment with these replacement ingredients and techniques to find the combination that best suits your taste and dietary needs. With a little creativity and a willingness to explore new options, you can create creamy tasting soups that taste extravagant but are in fact healthy and nutritious.

CHAPTER 6

· ·

TIME-SAVING TIPS FOR MAKING DELICIOUS SOUPS

Whether you're whipping up a hearty stew, a creamy bisque, or a light vegetable soup, it's essential to have a few time-saving tricks up your sleeve to make the whole process more efficient. These top tips will help you create flavorful soups without having to spend hours in the kitchen.

1. Prep Ahead of Time: Before you start cooking, take a few minutes to prep your ingredients. Chop vegetables, measure out spices, and have everything ready to go and close to hand. This will streamline the cooking process and prevent you from scrambling for ingredients as you cook.

2. Keep a Well-Stocked Pantry: Maintain a pantry stocked with canned legumes, lentils, pasta, rice, and other staples. Canned chopped tomatoes and potatoes are useful too. These ingredients can be the base for a variety of quick and satisfying soups.

3. Use Frozen Vegetables: Frozen vegetables are a time-saving wonder. They're already cleaned, chopped, and ready to use. Keep a variety of frozen veggies on hand to add to your soups for extra flavor and nutrition.

4. Choose Canned Broth or Stock: While homemade broth or stock is fantastic and if you have the time or inclination, is the best option for sure, but using canned or boxed versions is absolutely fine and will significantly cut down on cooking and prep time. Look for low-sodium options and enhance the flavor with your own choice of herbs and seasonings. But if you do want to make your own, I have included a method in a previous chapter.

5. Double the Recipe: When making soups, it often takes just a little extra effort to make a bigger batch and double the recipe. Freeze the extra portions for future meals, saving you time on cooking in the long run and this way, you'll have homemade soup on hand whenever you need a quick and convenient meal.

6. Utilize Pressure Cookers and Slow Cookers: Pressure cookers, like Instant Pots, can drastically reduce cooking times while infusing deep flavors into your soups. Whereas slow cookers are perfect for "set it and forget it" soups that simmer all day while you're busy.

7. Embrace One-Pot Meals: Luckily most of the recipes here are one-pot wonders, where you can cook everything in a single pot or pan. Fewer dishes mean less mess and cleaning-up and more time saved.

8. Repurpose Leftovers: Don't let leftover vegetables or proteins go to waste. Use them in your soups to add depth and flavor. For instance, leftover roasted chicken can become a hearty chicken noodle soup, and roasted veggies can enhance a vegetable medley soup.

9. Use Pre-Cut Herbs and Spices: While fresh herbs are lovely, pre-cut, and frozen herbs can be a really convenient alternative. They can be easily added to your soup without the need for chopping and measuring.

10. Consider Quick-Cooking Proteins: Choose proteins like shrimp, thinly sliced beef, or ground turkey that cook quickly. This way, you can have a protein-rich soup ready in no time.

With these time-saving tips, making delicious soups can be a breeze. Whether you're preparing a simple weeknight dinner or hosting a gathering, these strategies will help you get a hot and satisfying bowl of soup on the table with less stress and more enjoyment.

CHAPTER 7

· ·

FREEZING SOUPS:
UNLOCKING THE SECRETS OF SOUP PRESERVATION

There's something incredibly satisfying about a hearty bowl of homemade soup. Soups have a way of warming the soul and bringing comfort to our tables. But what happens when you make a big batch of soup and have more than you can eat in one go? That's where freezing comes to the rescue!

Why Freeze Soup?

Freezing soup is a fantastic way to extend the life of your culinary creations. It allows you to enjoy your favorite soups on busy weeknights or during those times when you simply don't feel like cooking from scratch. Plus, it helps reduce food waste by preserving leftovers. Here are a few reasons why freezing soup is a good idea:

Convenience: Having frozen soup on hand means you're just a quick thaw and reheat away from a delicious, homemade meal.

Preserve Freshness: Freezing soup locks in the flavors and nutrients, preserving the freshness of the ingredients.

Seasonal Ingredients: Capture the flavors of seasonal produce in soups and enjoy them throughout the rest of the year.

Reduce Food Waste: Prevent leftover soup from going to waste by freezing it for later consumption.

Emergency Meals: Frozen soups are perfect for those times when unexpected guests arrive or you're too ill or tired to cook.

Choosing the Right Containers

Before diving into the freezing process, it's important to choose what to put your soup in. The ideal container for freezing soup should be airtight, freezer-safe, and resistant to both extreme cold and heat. Here are some options:

Plastic Containers: Use BPA-free plastic containers with tight-fitting lids. Choose containers with airtight seals to prevent freezer burn.

Glass Containers: Heat-resistant glass containers with airtight lids are a great option. Just be sure to leave some space at the top for expansion.

Zip-Top Freezer Bags: These are space-saving and work well for liquid-based soups. Sit the bag in a rigid container and ¾ fill with soup. Squeeze out excess air before sealing.

Vacuum-Sealed Bags: If you have a vacuum sealer, it's an excellent way to remove air and prevent freezer burn.

Ice Cube Trays: Perfect for freezing smaller stock pot sized portions or for adding as a base to other soup dishes.

Proper Freezing Techniques

Now that you have your containers ready, it's time to freeze your soup properly. Follow these steps for successful soup preservation:

Cool Completely: Allow your soup to cool to room temperature before attempting to freeze it. Hot soup can raise the temperature in your freezer and harm other frozen items.

Portion Control: Decide how you want to portion your soup. You can freeze it in individual servings or in larger containers for family meals. Use labels, stickers, or permanent markers to note the date and type of soup.

Leave Room for Expansion: Liquids expand when frozen, so always leave a little space at the top to avoid spills or cracked containers.

Air Removal: If using airtight containers, press plastic wrap or parchment paper directly onto the surface of the soup before sealing the container. This minimizes its exposure to air and reduces the chance of freezer burn.

Labelling: Label each container with the type of soup and the date it was prepared. This helps you keep track of what's in your freezer and ensures you use the oldest soups first. Soup should be stored for a maximum of 3 months in the freezer.

Stack Smart: If you're using containers, stack them neatly in your freezer to maximize space. Remember, soups with different flavors or ingredients should be stored separately.

Thawing and Reheating

When you're ready to enjoy your frozen soup, you have a few options for thawing and reheating:

Refrigerator Thaw: Place the frozen container of soup in the refrigerator overnight. This slow thawing method ensures even heating when you're ready to enjoy it.

Stovetop Reheating: Transfer the thawed soup to a pot and heat it gently on the stove over a low to medium heat. Stir occasionally to prevent sticking or burning.

Microwave Re-heating: Use a microwave-safe dish, and heat the soup in 1-2 minute intervals, stirring between each interval until the soup is completely heated through.

Instant Pot or Slow Cooker: Use these kitchen appliances to reheat frozen soup safely and evenly.

Remember that soup stored in the freezer can typically last for 2-3 months, but for the best quality, try to consume it within the first month.

Freezing soup is a simple yet highly effective way to preserve the delicious flavors of your homemade creations. With the right containers, proper freezing techniques, and a bit of planning, you can ensure that a warm and satisfying bowl of soup is never too far from reach when you need it the most. So go ahead, make that extra batch of your favorite soup, and freeze it for future enjoyment.

CHAPTER 8

. . . .

SEASONING ALTERNATIVES

Seasonings are the soul of any dish, adding depth, flavor, and personality to every mouthful. While salt and pepper are the classics, the world of seasoning is vast and diverse, offering a treasure trove of alternatives to elevate your culinary creations. Whether you're looking to reduce your sodium intake, experiment with new flavors, or cater to specific dietary needs, there are plenty of different ways of seasoning to explore. Here are a few great ideas:

Herbaceous Wonders: Fresh and dried herbs are nature's gift to the culinary world. Basil, thyme, rosemary, and oregano can infuse your dishes with aromatic freshness. Chopped cilantro and parsley bring vibrant color and zesty notes. Experiment with a medley of herbs to find your perfect combination.

Spices Galore: Spices are the heart of global cuisine. From cumin and coriander to turmeric and paprika, spices offer a world of flavor. Dive into the rich tapestry of Indian, Middle Eastern, or Mexican spices to add complexity to your dishes.

Citrus Zest: The zest of lemons, limes, and oranges adds a burst of brightness to your meals. Grated citrus peel not only infuses dishes with vibrant flavors but also contributes a delightful texture.

Garlic and Onion Magic: Fresh or roasted garlic cloves, garlic powder, and onion powder are indispensable in the kitchen. They impart savory, umami-rich notes to your dishes, enhancing both the aroma and taste.

Heat with Peppers: If you crave heat, explore the world of chili peppers. Crushed red pepper flakes, cayenne pepper, and chipotle or ancho powder can bring the fire you're after. For a milder kick, consider paprika or sweet pepper blends.

Seeds and Nuts: Sesame seeds, poppy seeds, and toasted nuts like almonds and pine nuts introduce delightful textures and nutty undertones to your dishes. They're also excellent as garnishes.

Umami-Boosting Ingredients: Soy sauce, miso paste, and fish sauce are umami-rich alternatives to salt. They're perfect for Asian-inspired soups or broths and can be used sparingly to build layers of flavor into most soups.

Dried Fruits: Dried fruits such as raisins, apricots, and cranberries provide a hint of sweetness that can balance savory soups perfectly.

Vinegar Varieties: Vinegars like balsamic, apple cider, and rice vinegar offer acidity and depth. The sharpness they add can really lift an average soup from tasty to delicious.

Freshness of Ginger: Freshly grated or minced ginger adds a zingy, spicy-sweet note to soups, and stews.

Dried Mushrooms: Dried porcini or shiitake mushrooms, when rehydrated and finely chopped, infuse dishes with a rich, earthy flavor reminiscent of umami.

Herb Blends: Experiment with herb blends like Italian seasoning, herbes de Provence, or za'atar, which are pre-mixed combinations of herbs and spices designed to elevate specific cuisines.

Smoked Ingredients: Smoked paprika, smoked salt, or liquid smoke can lend a smoky depth to vegetarian or vegan soups, replicating the flavors of grilling or smoking.

Nutritional Yeast: This vegan-friendly ingredient provides a cheesy, nutty flavor that's perfect for dairy-free recipes or those needing a tasty boost.

By exploring these seasoning alternatives, you can ensure that your creations don't lack taste. As with most elements of cooking, you'll only get better by trying different things and using alternative seasonings is a great way to do this.

CHAPTER 9

. . . .

A QUICK NOTE ON COOKING GARLIC

You may be wondering why I would dedicate a whole section to cooking garlic? Well, that's because it appears in almost every recipe in the book along with other soup staples like onions, celery, and carrots. But unlike all those other ingredients, garlic can easily be ruined, and with that comes a change in taste which we don't want.

So be creative and artistic with your soup making, but make sure you at least give garlic the attention that it needs

Cooking garlic correctly is an essential skill for any home chef, as it can elevate the flavor of a wide variety of dishes. Garlic, known for its pungent aroma and savory taste, is a versatile ingredient that can be used in countless recipes. To get the best out of garlic, it's important to know how to cook it correctly. Here's a step-by-step description of how to do just that:

1. Select Fresh Garlic: Start by choosing fresh garlic bulbs with firm, unblemished cloves. Avoid garlic bulbs that feel soft or have sprouted, as they may be past their prime.

2. Peel the Garlic: To use garlic in your recipes, you'll need to remove the papery skin. There are a few methods to peel garlic cloves effectively. One common method is to place the flat side of a chef's knife on a garlic clove and press down firmly until it crushes slightly. This makes it easier to peel away the skin. Alternatively, you can place the garlic cloves in a container, like a small glass jar, and shake vigorously; the skins will loosen, making them easier to peel.

3. Choose Your Cooking Method: There are various ways to cook garlic, and the method you choose depends on the flavor you want to achieve. Here are a few popular methods:

Minced or Chopped Garlic: Finely chopping or mincing garlic is a common method. It's great for evenly distributing garlic flavor throughout a dish. Use a sharp knife and a rocking motion to mince the garlic finely.

Sliced Garlic: Sliced garlic adds a milder garlic flavor. Slice the garlic cloves thinly using a sharp knife.

Whole Garlic Cloves: Roasting whole garlic cloves in their skin can yield a sweet, mellow garlic flavor. Simply toss them in olive oil and roast until they're soft and caramelized or bake in their skins in a moderate oven for 10 minutes.

Crushed or Smashed Garlic: Crushing or smashing garlic cloves releases more of its pungent oils and flavors. Use the flat side of a knife or a garlic press for this method. Crushed garlic is excellent for infusing into oils and sauces.

4. Control the Heat: When cooking garlic, it's important to control the heat to avoid burning it, which can result in a bitter taste. Start by heating your pan over low-medium heat and add oil or butter. Once it's hot, add your garlic. Sauté the garlic for about 30 seconds to 1 minute, stirring constantly until it becomes fragrant and only slightly golden. Be vigilant; garlic can go from golden to burnt very quickly indeed!

5. Experiment with Roasting: Roasting garlic is a wonderful way to bring out its sweet, nutty flavor. To roast garlic bulbs, cut off the top portion to expose the cloves, drizzle with olive oil, wrap in foil, and bake in the oven until soft and caramelized. The roasted cloves can be squeezed out and used as a spread or added to dishes.

Learning how to cook garlic correctly can enhance the taste of your soups. Whether you prefer the bold punch of minced garlic or the subtle sweetness of roasted garlic, using these techniques will open up a world of flavor possibilities in your cooking.

GLOSSARY OF TERMS

Shredded: Shredded refers to food items that have been cut or torn into long, thin strips or threads. This technique is often used for vegetables like cabbage or carrots and can also apply to meats and cheeses.

Chopped: Chopped signifies that ingredients have been cut into smaller, irregular pieces. The size of the pieces can vary depending on the recipe, but typically they are larger than minced or diced pieces.

Smashed: Smashed describes the action of pressing down on food items, often with a utensil like a fork or a masher, to flatten or break them into smaller, less uniform pieces. This technique is frequently used for potatoes or garlic cloves.

Cubed: Cubed ingredients have been cut into uniformly sized, cube-shaped pieces. The size of the cubes can vary, ranging from small cubes for precision in cooking to larger ones for stews and soups.

Peeled: Peeled refers to the removal of the outer skin or peel from fruits or vegetables. This process is usually done using a knife or a peeler to reveal the edible flesh beneath.

Charred: Charred indicates that food items have been exposed to high heat, often an open flame or a hot surface, until they develop a dark, slightly burnt, or caramelized exterior. This technique can add a smoky or charred flavor to the dish.

Diced: Diced ingredients have been cut into small, uniform cubes. This technique results in pieces that are smaller than those typically achieved through chopping.

Sauté: Sautéing involves cooking food quickly in a small amount of oil or butter over a high heat. It's a method used to brown the ingredients while preserving their texture and flavor.

Minced: Minced ingredients have been finely chopped into very small, uniform pieces. This technique is often used for herbs, garlic, and other aromatics to release their essential flavors.

Crushed: Crushed signifies that food items have been pressed, pounded, or otherwise broken down into smaller pieces, often with the intention of releasing their natural juices or flavors.

Julienne: Julienning vegetables is a culinary technique that involves cutting vegetables into long, thin, matchstick-like strips. This method not only adds an elegant touch to your dishes but also helps vegetables cook quickly and evenly.

Broth: Broth is a savory liquid that is made from simmering meats, vegetables, or bones in water. It serves as the base for soups, stews, and sauces and can be seasoned with herbs and spices for added flavor.

Ok, that's most of the housekeeping out of the way, there's just a few more tips for you and general cooking advice at the back of the book.

Now let's move onto the actual recipes. You'll find over 100 different recipes (105 to be precise!) and they have been split into the following sections:

- BEEF SOUP RECIPES
- PORK SOUP RECIPES
- CHICKEN SOUP RECIPES
- SEAFOOD SOUP RECIPES
- FISH SOUP RECIPES
- VEGETARIAN SOUP RECIPES
- VEGAN SOUP RECIPES

Now, many of these recipes are interchangeable, so for example if you see a beef-based soup that you like the look of, then there's absolutely no reason why you can't substitute the beef with chicken, mushrooms, or fish for example.

I've included an approximate calorie count for each soup, although this should only be taken as a guide, not an exact measure as there can be a big difference between ingredients. An example of this would be shop bought beef broth which may contain much less or far more calories than a home-made version, or certain cuts of meats etc.

Also, I've included the recipes for most of these soups in larger quantities so there is enough for between 4-6 portions. But, if you don't want to make that much and freeze or refrigerate for use over the next few days, then you should reduce the quantities in the ingredients section and simply make less.

Alost every recipe calls for the use of broth (stock) and these are widely available at supermarkets in jars, bottles, or boxes. There are basically a couple of options:

Shop-bought stock, either in the form of cubes, bouillon powder or fresh stock in the refrigerated section of your local supermarket or homemade stock. The easiest and cheapest way of doing this is by using stock or broth cubes instead and adding it to the stated amount of water.

Making the soup thinner or thicker: It's a really good idea to take out some of the soup liquid before blending, by skimming off the top of the pot. You can then add back after blending if the texture of the soup is too thick. If you blend it all in one go, there's a chance it might be too thin for your liking, so this way you can get the exact texture you prefer.

I think that's most things covered, I hope you find some recipes that you like and make on a regular basis, but don't be too regimented about it, you should change the recipe to your own individual taste and preference. Remember the only limit to soup making is your imagination!

BEEF
SOUP
RECIPES

CLASSIC BEEF VEGETABLE SOUP

SERVINGS: 6 | CALORIES PER SERVING: 195KCAL | TOTAL COOKING TIME: 40 MINS

INGREDIENTS

- 1 lb lean ground beef
- 1 onion, chopped
- 2 carrots, peeled and diced
- 2 celery stalks, diced
- 2 garlic cloves, minced
- 4 cups low-sodium beef or vegetable broth
- 1 can (14 oz/400g) diced tomatoes
- 2 potatoes, peeled and diced into small pieces
- 1 cup green beans, trimmed and cut into bite-sized pieces
- 1 cup corn kernels (fresh, frozen, or canned)
- 1 tsp dried thyme
- 1 tsp dried oregano
- Salt and pepper to taste
- 2 cups baby spinach or kale, chopped
- Fresh parsley, chopped (for garnish)

METHOD

1. In a large pot or Dutch oven, cook the lean ground beef over medium heat until browned. Use a wooden spoon to break it into smaller pieces as it cooks. Once cooked, remove any excess fat.

2. Add the chopped onion, diced carrots, and diced celery to the pot. Cook for about 5 minutes, or until the vegetables start to soften.

3. Add the minced garlic and cook for an additional 1-2 minutes, until fragrant.

4. Pour in the low-sodium beef or vegetable broth and the can of diced tomatoes (with their juice). Stir to combine.

5. Add the diced potatoes, green beans, and corn kernels to the pot. Stir in the dried thyme and dried oregano. Season with salt and pepper to taste.

6. Bring the soup to a boil, then reduce the heat to low. Cover the pot and let the soup simmer for about 20-25 minutes, or until the vegetables are tender.

7. Just before serving, stir in the chopped baby spinach or kale. The heat of the soup will wilt the greens.

8. Taste the soup and adjust the seasoning if needed.

9. Ladle the hot beef vegetable soup into bowls. Garnish with fresh chopped parsley.

10. Serve the soup with whole-grain bread or rolls for a complete and satisfying meal.

BEEF AND BARLEY SOUP

SERVINGS: 6 | CALORIES PER SERVING: 200KCAL | TOTAL COOKING TIME: 65 MINS

INGREDIENTS

1 lb lean beef stew meat, cubed

1 cup pearl barley

1 onion, chopped

2 carrots, peeled and chopped

3 cloves garlic, minced

8 cups low-sodium beef or vegetable broth

1 bay leaf

1 tsp dried thyme

1 tsp dried rosemary

1 tsp paprika

Salt and pepper to taste

2 tbsp olive oil

Fresh parsley, chopped (for garnish)

METHOD

1. Heat the olive oil in a large soup pot over medium heat. Add the beef cubes and cook until browned on all sides. Remove the beef from the pot and set aside.

2. In the same pot, add the chopped onion, and carrots. Sauté for about 5 minutes, or until the vegetables begin to soften.

3. Add the minced garlic, dried thyme, dried rosemary, and paprika to the pot. Sauté for an additional 1-2 minutes, until fragrant.

4. Return the browned beef cubes to the pot. Add the pearl barley and bay leaf.

5. Pour in the low-sodium beef or vegetable broth. Bring the mixture to a boil, then reduce the heat to low. Cover the pot and let the soup simmer for about 45-50 minutes, or until the beef is tender and the barley is cooked.

6. Season the soup with salt and pepper to taste. Remember that low-sodium broth already contains some salt, so adjust according to your preference.

7. Once the soup is cooked and the flavors have blended, remove the bay leaf from the pot.

8. Ladle the soup into serving bowls. Garnish each bowl with chopped fresh parsley for added color and flavor.

9. Serve hot, accompanied by crusty whole-grain bread or a side salad.

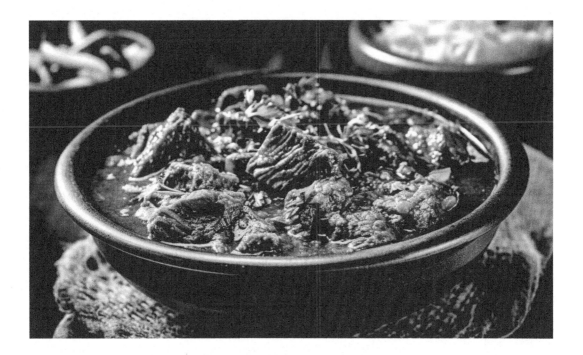

You can make this recipe your own by adding more vegetables like peas, green beans, or spinach for added nutrition. You can also use a slow cooker for a more convenient cooking process.

BEEF AND LENTIL SOUP

SERVINGS: 6 | CALORIES PER SERVING: 170KCAL | TOTAL COOKING TIME: 50 MINS

INGREDIENTS

1   lb lean ground beef

1   cup dried green or brown lentils, rinsed and drained

1   onion, chopped

2   carrots, peeled and chopped

3   cloves garlic, minced

6   cups low-sodium beef or vegetable broth

1   can (14 oz/400g) diced tomatoes

1   tsp dried thyme

1   tsp dried rosemary

1   tsp ground cumin

1   bay leaf

    Salt and pepper to taste

METHOD

1. In a large pot or Dutch oven, brown the lean ground beef over medium heat until cooked through. Break it into smaller pieces as it cooks. Once cooked, remove any excess fat.

2. Add the chopped onion, and carrots, to the pot. Sauté for about 5 minutes, until the vegetables start to soften.

3. Stir in the minced garlic, dried thyme, dried rosemary, and ground cumin. Cook for another minute until fragrant.

4. Add the rinsed lentils to the pot and give everything a good stir.

5. Pour in the low-sodium beef or vegetable broth and the can of diced tomatoes (with their juice). Add the bay leaf. Stir to combine.

6. Bring the soup to a boil, then reduce the heat to low. Cover the pot and let the soup simmer for about 25-30 minutes, or until the lentils are tender.

7. Season the soup with salt and pepper to taste. Keep in mind that if you're using store-bought broth, it may already contain some salt, so adjust accordingly.

8. Remove the bay leaf from the soup.

9. Ladle the soup into bowls and garnish with fresh chopped parsley.

FRENCH ONION SOUP WITH BEEF

SERVINGS: 6 | CALORIES PER SERVING: 400KCAL | TOTAL COOKING TIME: 90 MINS

INGREDIENTS

For the Soup:

2   tbsp olive oil

2   pounds (900g) lean beef stew meat, cubed into bite sized pieces

4   large onions, thinly sliced

4   cloves garlic, minced

6   cups low-sodium beef broth

2   cups water

2   bay leaves

1   tsp dried thyme

    Salt and black pepper to taste

For the Topping:

    Whole grain baguette slices

1   cup reduced-fat Swiss or Gruyere cheese, shredded

This version of French Onion Soup uses lean beef and reduced-fat cheese for a healthier twist on the classic recipe. It's still flavorful and satisfying while being mindful of nutritional goals.

METHOD

1. Heat the olive oil in a large pot over medium-high heat. Add the beef cubes and brown them on all sides. Remove the beef from the pot and set it aside.

2. In the same pot, add the sliced onions and sauté until they start to caramelize -about 15-20 minutes.

3. Add the minced garlic and sauté for an additional 1-2 minutes until fragrant.

4. Return the browned beef to the pot and add the beef broth, water, bay leaves, dried thyme, salt, and black pepper. Bring the mixture to a simmer.

5. Reduce the heat to low, cover the pot, and let the soup simmer for about an hour, or until the beef is tender.

6. While the soup is simmering and nearly cooked, preheat the oven to broil. Place the whole grain baguette slices on a baking sheet and toast them in the oven until they are lightly browned.

7. Once the soup is ready, discard the bay leaves. Taste and adjust the seasoning if needed.

8. Preheat the broiler again. Ladle the soup into oven-safe bowls.

9. Place a toasted baguette slice on top of each bowl of soup and sprinkle a generous amount of reduced-fat Swiss or Gruyere cheese on top.

10. Place the bowls under the broiler until the cheese is melted and bubbly, about 2-3 minutes. Keep a close eye on it to avoid burning.

11. Carefully remove the bowls from the oven using oven mitts.

12. Allow the soup to cool slightly before serving.

SPICY BEEF TORTILLA SOUP

SERVINGS: 6 | CALORIES PER SERVING: 235KCAL | TOTAL COOKING TIME: 35 MINS

INGREDIENTS

1   lb lean ground beef

1   onion, chopped

3   cloves garlic, minced

1   bell pepper, diced

1   jalapeño pepper, minced (adjust to taste)

1   can (14 oz/400g) diced tomatoes

1   can (14 oz/400g) black beans, drained and rinsed

1   cup frozen corn kernels

6   cups low-sodium beef or vegetable broth

1   tsp chili powder

1   tsp cumin

½   tsp smoked paprika

Salt and pepper to taste

1 tbsp olive oil

For Serving:

Baked tortilla strips or tortilla chips

Fresh cilantro, chopped

Lime wedges

Avocado slices

Fat-free Greek yogurt or sour cream (optional)

METHOD

1. Heat a large pot over medium heat. Add the olive oil, then add the lean ground beef. Cook, breaking it up with a spoon, until browned. Remove any excess fat if needed.

2. Add the chopped onion, diced bell pepper, minced jalapeño, and minced garlic to the pot. Sauté for a 2-3 minutes until the vegetables are softened.

3. Stir in the chili powder, cumin, smoked paprika, salt, and pepper. Cook for another minute until the spices are fragrant.

4. Add the diced tomatoes, black beans, and frozen corn kernels to the pot. Stir to combine.

5. Pour in the low-sodium beef or vegetable broth. Bring the soup to a boil, then reduce the heat to a simmer. Let the soup simmer for about 15-20 minutes to allow the flavors to blend.

6. Taste and adjust the seasoning if needed. If you prefer a milder soup, you can reduce the amount of jalapeño or omit it altogether.

7. While the soup is simmering, prepare your toppings. Cut corn tortillas into thin strips and bake them in the oven until crispy for a healthier alternative to traditional fried tortilla strips.

8. Serve the soup hot in bowls. Top each serving with baked tortilla strips, chopped fresh cilantro, a squeeze of lime juice, avocado slices, and a dollop of fat-free Greek yogurt or sour cream if desired.

BEEF AND CABBAGE SOUP

SERVINGS: 6 | CALORIES PER SERVING: 150KCAL | TOTAL COOKING TIME: 40 MINS

INGREDIENTS

1   tbsp olive oil
1   lb (450g) lean ground beef
1   onion, diced
2   cloves garlic, minced
4   cups beef broth
    (low sodium)
2   cups water
2   cups cabbage, shredded
2   carrots, peeled and sliced
2   celery stalks, sliced
1   can (14 oz/400g) diced
    tomatoes (no salt added)
1   tsp dried thyme
1   tsp dried oregano
1   bay leaf
    Salt and pepper to taste
    Fresh parsley, chopped
    (for garnish)

METHOD

1. In a large pot or Dutch oven, heat a drizzle of olive oil over medium heat. Add the lean ground beef and cook until browned. Break it up with a spoon as it cooks.

2. Add diced onion and minced garlic to the pot with the ground beef. Sauté for a few minutes until the onion becomes translucent.

3. Pour in the beef broth and water. Stir to combine.

4. Add the shredded cabbage, sliced carrots, and celery to the pot.

5. Drain the can of diced tomatoes and add them to the pot.

6. Stir in the dried thyme, dried oregano, and bay leaf.

7. Season the soup with a pinch of salt and a dash of black pepper. Remember that the beef broth might already contain some salt, so adjust to your taste.

8. Bring the soup to a boil, then reduce the heat to low. Cover the pot and let the soup simmer for about 20-25 minutes, or until the vegetables are tender.

9. Taste and adjust the seasoning if needed.

10. Once the soup is ready, remove the bay leaf and discard it.

11. Serve the beef and cabbage soup hot, garnished with chopped fresh parsley.

BEEF NOODLE SOUP

SERVINGS: 6 | CALORIES PER SERVING: 350KCAL | TOTAL COOKING TIME: 60 MINS

INGREDIENTS

For the Broth:

8 cups beef broth (low sodium)

1 onion, sliced

3 cloves garlic, minced

1-inch piece of ginger, sliced

2 carrots, peeled and sliced

1 star anise (optional)

1 cinnamon stick (optional)

Salt and pepper to taste

For the Soup:

8 oz lean beef (such as sirloin), thinly sliced

4 oz rice noodles or whole wheat noodles

2 cups baby spinach or bok choy

1 cup bean sprouts

2 green onions, sliced

Fresh cilantro leaves for garnish

Lime wedges for serving

1 sliced red chilli for serving

METHOD

1. In a large pot, add the beef broth, sliced onion, minced garlic, ginger, and carrots. If using, add the star anise and cinnamon stick for flavor. Season with a pinch of salt and pepper. Bring the broth to a simmer over medium heat and let it cook for about 20-30 minutes to develop the flavors.

2. Once the broth has simmered and the vegetables are tender, strain the broth through a fine mesh strainer or cheesecloth to remove the solids. Return the clear broth to the pot and discard the solids.

3. Cook the rice noodles or whole wheat noodles according to the package instructions. Drain and set aside.

4. Season the thinly sliced beef with a pinch of salt and pepper. In a separate skillet, heat a small amount of oil over medium-high heat. Add the beef slices and quickly sear them until they are browned on the outside but still slightly pink inside. Remove from heat and set aside.

5. Divide the cooked noodles among serving bowls. Top with baby spinach or bok choy, bean sprouts, and green onions.

6. Carefully ladle the hot strained broth over the noodles and vegetables in each bowl. The hot broth will cook the vegetables slightly.

7. Divide the seared beef slices among the bowls, placing them on top of the vegetables.

8. Garnish each bowl with fresh cilantro leaves and a lime wedge. The lime can be squeezed into the soup just before eating to add a burst of flavor.

9. Serve the beef noodle soup immediately while it's still hot. Squeeze lime over the soup just before eating for added freshness and tanginess.

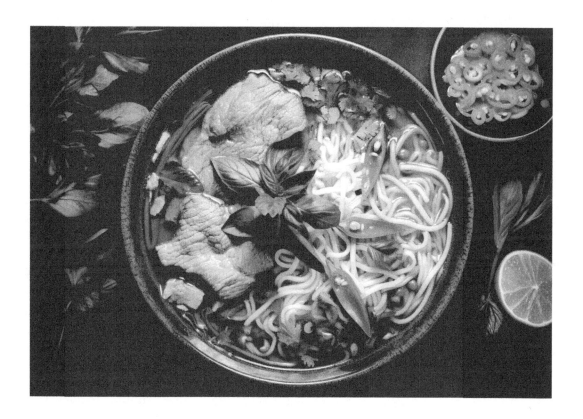

BEEF AND MUSHROOM SOUP

SERVINGS: 6 | CALORIES PER SERVING: 200KCAL | TOTAL COOKING TIME: 45 MINS

INGREDIENTS

- 1 lb lean beef (such as sirloin or stew meat), thinly sliced
- 1 cup mushrooms, sliced
- 1 onion, finely chopped
- 2 carrots, peeled and diced
- 3 cloves garlic, minced
- 6 cups low-sodium beef or vegetable broth
- 1 tsp dried thyme
- 1 tsp dried rosemary
- 1 bay leaf
- Salt and pepper to taste
- 2 tbsp olive oil
- Fresh parsley, chopped (for garnish)

METHOD

1. Heat a large pot or Dutch oven over medium heat. Add the olive oil and allow it to heat up.
2. Add the sliced beef to the pot and cook until browned on all sides. Remove the beef from the pot and set it aside.
3. In the same pot, add the chopped onion and sauté for about 2-3 minutes until it becomes translucent.
4. Add the minced garlic, and diced carrots to the pot. Sauté for an additional 3-4 minutes.
5. Add the sliced mushrooms to the pot and cook for another 3-4 minutes until they start to soften.
6. Return the browned beef to the pot and mix it with the vegetables.
7. Pour in the beef or vegetable broth and stir to combine.
8. Add the dried thyme, dried rosemary, bay leaf, and season with salt and pepper to taste. Stir to incorporate the herbs and spices.
9. Bring the soup to a boil, then reduce the heat to low. Cover the pot and let the soup simmer for about 20-25 minutes to allow the flavors to blend together.
10. Taste the soup and adjust the seasoning if needed.
11. Remove the bay leaf from the soup and discard.
12. Ladle the soup into bowls and garnish with chopped fresh parsley.
13. Serve the soup hot with whole-grain bread or a side salad for a complete and satisfying meal.

You can customize this recipe by adding other vegetables like peas or spinach for extra nutrients.

BEEF AND VEGETABLE MINESTRONE

SERVINGS: 6 | CALORIES PER SERVING: 265KCAL | TOTAL COOKING TIME: 40 MINS

INGREDIENTS

1   lb lean ground beef

1   onion, chopped

2   carrots, peeled and diced

3   garlic cloves, minced

1   zucchini, diced

1   yellow bell pepper, diced

1   can (14 oz/400g) diced tomatoes

6   cups low-sodium beef or vegetable broth

1   cup cooked kidney beans (canned or cooked from dry)

1   cup cooked whole wheat pasta (such as macaroni or small shells)

1   tsp dried oregano

1   tsp dried basil

½   tsp dried thyme

   Salt and pepper to taste

2   cups baby spinach or kale, chopped

   Grated Parmesan cheese (optional, for serving)

   Fresh chopped parsley (for garnish)

   Olive oil (for cooking)

METHOD

1. In a large pot or Dutch oven, heat a drizzle of olive oil over medium heat. Add the lean ground beef and cook until browned. Break it up with a spoon as it cooks. Once cooked, transfer the beef to a plate and set aside.

2. In the same pot, add a bit more olive oil if needed. Add the chopped onion, diced carrots, and minced garlic. Sauté for a few minutes until the vegetables start to soften.

3. Add the diced zucchini and yellow bell pepper to the pot. Cook for a few more minutes until the vegetables are slightly tender.

4. Return the cooked ground beef to the pot. Add the can of diced tomatoes (with juice), dried oregano, dried basil, dried thyme, salt, and pepper. Stir to combine the flavors.

5. Pour in the beef or vegetable broth and bring the soup to a simmer. Let it cook for about 15-20 minutes to allow the flavors to blend together.

6. Add the cooked kidney beans and cooked whole wheat pasta to the pot. Stir to combine and let the soup simmer for another 5-10 minutes.

7. Just before serving, stir in the chopped baby spinach or kale. Let it wilt into the soup.

8. Taste and adjust the seasoning with more salt and pepper if needed.

9. Ladle the minestrone into serving bowls. If desired, sprinkle some grated Parmesan cheese on top of each bowl.

10. Garnish with freshly chopped parsley for a burst of freshness just before serving.

THAI BEEF COCONUT SOUP

SERVINGS: 4 | CALORIES PER SERVING: 300KCAL | TOTAL COOKING TIME: 30 MINS

INGREDIENTS

2 cups low-sodium beef or vegetable broth

1 can (14 oz/400g) coconut milk

2 stalks lemongrass, bruised and cut into 2-inch pieces

3-4 slices galangal (Thai ginger) or regular ginger

3-4 kaffir lime leaves, torn into pieces

2-3 Thai bird's eye chilies, lightly crushed (adjust to taste)

3 cloves garlic, minced

1 small onion, thinly sliced

1 cup sliced mushrooms (such as button or shiitake)

1 medium carrot, thinly sliced

1 red bell pepper, sliced

1 cup sliced cooked beef (such as steak or roast beef)

1 tbsp coconut oil or cooking oil

2 tbsp fish sauce (adjust to taste)

1 tbsp soy sauce (optional, for additional flavor)

1 tbsp lime juice

1 tsp brown sugar (optional, to balance flavors)

Salt and pepper to taste

Fresh cilantro leaves and chopped green onions for garnish

METHOD

1. Bruise the lemongrass stalks by gently pounding them with the back of a knife or rolling pin to release the flavor, slice the galangal into thin slices and tear the kaffir lime leaves to release their aroma. Thinly slice the onion, carrot, red bell pepper, and cooked beef.

2. In a soup pot, heat the coconut oil over medium heat, then add minced garlic and sliced onions. Sauté until the onions are translucent and fragrant.

3. Pour in the low-sodium beef or vegetable broth and coconut milk. Stir to combine.

4. Add the bruised lemongrass, galangal slices, torn kaffir lime leaves, and lightly crushed Thai bird's eye chilies to the pot. Bring the mixture to a gentle simmer. Let it simmer for about 10 minutes to infuse the flavors.

5. Add the sliced mushrooms, carrot, red bell pepper, and sliced cooked beef and stir gently.

6. Stir in fish sauce, soy sauce (if using), lime juice, and brown sugar (if desired). Adjust the seasonings according to your taste preferences.

7. Allow the soup to simmer for an additional 5-7 minutes, or until the vegetables are tender and the flavors are well combined.

8. Taste the soup and adjust the seasoning as needed. You can add more fish sauce, lime juice, or a pinch of salt and pepper if desired.

9. Ladle into serving bowls and garnish with fresh cilantro leaves and chopped green onions.

This soup is also known as "Tom Kha Gai." It offers a balance of flavors, from the creaminess of coconut milk to the aromatic spices and the tender slices of beef and vegetables. It pairs well with steamed rice or rice noodles if you prefer a heartier dish.

Start with a Good Base: Use a flavorful broth or stock as the foundation for your soup.

Fresh Ingredients: Use fresh, high-quality vegetables and meats for the best taste.

Sauté Aromatics: Onions, garlic, and other aromatics sautéed in oil create a flavor base.

VIETNAMESE PHO

SERVINGS: 6 | CALORIES PER SERVING: 300KCAL | TOTAL COOKING TIME: 70 MINS

INGREDIENTS

For the Broth:

2 medium onions, peeled halved and charred

3-inch piece of ginger, halved and charred

4-5 star anise

4-5 cloves

1 cinnamon stick

1 tsp coriander seeds

8 cups low-sodium beef or vegetable broth

1 tbsp low-sodium soy sauce or tamari

1 tbsp fish sauce (optional)

Salt and pepper, to taste

For the Soup:

8 oz rice noodles (Pho noodles)

8 oz cooked lean beef

Bean sprouts, for serving

Fresh herbs (Thai basil, cilantro, mint), for serving

Lime wedges, for serving

Sliced fresh chili peppers or Sriracha sauce, for serving

Hoisin sauce (optional), for serving

METHOD

1. Place the halved onions and ginger on a baking sheet and char them under the broiler or over an open flame until they are slightly blackened and fragrant. This step adds depth to the broth's flavor.

2. In a dry pan, toast the star anise, cloves, cinnamon stick, and coriander seeds over medium heat until fragrant. This step also enhances the broth's aroma.

3. In a large pot, add the toasted spices, charred onions, charred ginger, beef or vegetable broth, soy sauce or tamari, and fish sauce (if using). Bring the mixture to a simmer and let it cook for about 30-40 minutes. Skim off any impurities that rise to the surface.

4. Strain the broth through a fine mesh sieve into another a large bowl. Discard the solids.

5. Cook the rice noodles according to the package instructions. Drain and rinse them under cold water to stop the cooking process and prevent them from becoming too soft.

6. Divide the cooked noodles among serving bowls. Top with the cooked lean beef.

7. Carefully ladle the hot broth over the noodles and protein. The hot broth will heat up the cooked protein and soften the noodles.

8. Serve the Pho bowls with a platter of fresh bean sprouts, Thai basil, cilantro, mint, lime wedges, sliced chili peppers or Sriracha sauce, and hoisin sauce on the side.

This recipe provides a healthy version of Vietnamese Pho that's packed with flavor, lean protein, and fresh herbs. You can adjust the ingredients to suit your dietary preferences and make it as spicy or as mild as you prefer.

BEEF TACO SOUP

• •

SERVINGS: 6 | CALORIES PER SERVING: 220KCAL | TOTAL COOKING TIME: 450 MINS

INGREDIENTS

1   lb lean ground beef (you can also use ground turkey or chicken)
1   onion, chopped
2   cloves garlic, minced
1   bell pepper, chopped
1   can (14 oz/400g) black beans, drained and rinsed
1   can (14 oz/400g) kidney beans, drained and rinsed
1   can (14 oz/400g) corn kernels, drained
1   can (14 oz/400g) diced tomatoes
1   can (4 oz/115g) diced green chilies
4   cups low-sodium beef or vegetable broth
1   packet low-sodium taco seasoning
1   tsp ground cumin
1   tsp chili powder
    Salt and pepper to taste

Optional toppings:
    chopped cilantro, sliced green onions, shredded cheese, fat free plain Greek yogurt or sour cream, avocado slices, lime wedges

METHOD

1. In a large soup pot or Dutch oven, cook the ground beef over medium-high heat until browned. Drain off any excess fat.

2. Add chopped onions, minced garlic, and chopped bell pepper to the pot. Cook for a few minutes until the vegetables start to soften.

3. Sprinkle the taco seasoning, ground cumin, and chili powder over the beef and vegetables. Stir well to coat everything with the seasoning.

4. Add the drained black beans, kidney beans, corn kernels, diced tomatoes, and diced green chilies to the pot. Stir to combine.

5. Pour in the low-sodium beef or vegetable broth. You can adjust the amount of broth based on how thick or soupy you prefer the soup.

6. Bring the soup to a simmer. Reduce the heat to low and let it simmer for about 15-20 minutes, allowing the flavors to blend together.

7. Taste the soup and add salt and pepper as needed. The taco seasoning might already contain salt, so adjust accordingly.

8. Ladle the soup into bowls. Garnish with your choice of toppings, such as chopped cilantro, sliced green onions, shredded cheese, plain Greek yogurt or sour cream, avocado slices, and a squeeze of lime juice.

9. Serve your delicious and healthy beef taco soup with whole-grain tortilla chips or a side of whole-grain bread.

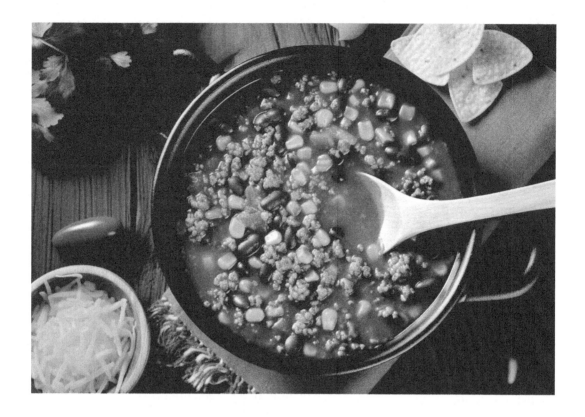

This beef taco soup is loaded with protein, fiber, and veggies, making it a nutritious and satisfying meal.

RUSSIAN BORSCHT

SERVINGS: 6 | CALORIES PER SERVING: 195KCAL | TOTAL COOKING TIME: 50 MINS

INGREDIENTS

For the Soup:

1 lb (450g) lean beef stew meat, cubed into bite sized pieces

1 onion, chopped

2 carrots, peeled and chopped

2 medium beets (beetroot), peeled and grated

2 potatoes, peeled and diced

2 cups cabbage, shredded

3 cloves garlic, minced

6 cups beef or vegetable broth

1 can (14 oz/400g) diced tomatoes

2 bay leaves

1 tsp dried thyme

Salt and pepper to taste

Olive oil for cooking

For the Sour Cream Topping:

1 cup fat free Greek yogurt or sour cream

Fresh dill, chopped, for garnish

Fresh parsley, chopped, for garnish

METHOD

1. Heat a large pot over medium-high heat. Add a drizzle of olive oil and sear the beef cubes until browned on all sides. Remove the beef from the pot and set aside.

2. In the same pot, add a bit more olive oil if needed. Sauté the chopped onion, carrots, and grated beets for 3-4 minutes until the vegetables begin to soften.

3. Stir in the minced garlic, dried thyme, bay leaves, salt, and pepper. Cook for about a minute until the garlic becomes fragrant.

4. Pour in the beef or vegetable broth and add the diced tomatoes (with their juice). Bring the mixture to a simmer.

5. Return the seared beef cubes to the pot. Cover and let the soup simmer gently for about 30 minutes, or until the beef is tender.

6. Add the diced potatoes and shredded cabbage to the pot. Continue to simmer for another 15-20 minutes until the potatoes are cooked through. Remove the bay leaves.

7. Taste the soup and adjust the seasoning with more salt and pepper if needed.

8. Ladle the hot borscht into bowls. If desired, garnish with chopped fresh dill and parsley.

9. In a small bowl, mix the fat-free Greek yogurt until smooth.

10. Serve the borscht with a dollop of Greek yogurt or sour cream on top. The sour cream adds creaminess and tanginess to the soup.

This recipe is a healthier take on traditional Russian Borscht. Using lean beef, plenty of vegetables, and fat-free Greek yogurt as a topping adds a nutritious twist to this classic dish. It is traditionally served with dark rye bread.

KOREAN BEEF SEAWEED SOUP

SERVINGS: 6 | CALORIES PER SERVING: 175KCAL | TOTAL COOKING TIME: 50 MINS

INGREDIENTS

- 1 oz dried miyeok (seaweed)
- 4 cups water
- 1 tbsp sesame oil
- 2 cloves garlic, minced
- ½ lb lean beef (flank steak or sirloin), thinly sliced
- 1 tbsp soy sauce
  Salt and pepper to taste
- 4 cups beef or vegetable broth
- 1 cup sliced mushrooms (shiitake or button mushrooms)
- 2 green onions, sliced
- 2 eggs, beaten
  Toasted sesame seeds, for garnish (optional)

Otherwise known as "Miyeokguk." This traditional Korean soup is both nourishing and delicious, it's rich in flavors, packed with protein, and provides the health benefits of seaweed, which is a good source of minerals and nutrients.

METHOD

1. Rinse the dried miyeok (seaweed) under cold water to remove any sand or impurities. Soak the seaweed in water for about 30 minutes or until it softens. Drain and cut it into bite-sized pieces.

2. In a pot, heat the sesame oil over medium heat. Add the minced garlic and sauté for about 1 minute until fragrant. Add the sliced beef and cook until it's no longer pink. Season with soy sauce, salt, and pepper.

3. Pour in the beef or vegetable broth and water, then bring the mixture to a boil. Add the soaked and cut miyeok (seaweed) to the pot and let it simmer for about 20-25 minutes until the seaweed is tender.

4. Add the sliced mushrooms to the soup and let them cook for an additional 5-7 minutes until they're tender.

5. Taste the soup and adjust the seasoning with salt and pepper if needed. Stir in most of the sliced green onions, reserving some for garnish.

6. Slowly pour the beaten eggs into the soup while gently stirring in a circular motion. The eggs will create ribbons as they cook in the hot broth.

7. Ladle the soup into bowls and garnish with the remaining sliced green onions and toasted sesame seeds, if desired.

8. Serve the soup hot as a nourishing and comforting meal. It's a traditional dish often enjoyed on birthdays and special occasions in Korean culture.

BEEF AND POTATO SOUP

• •

SERVINGS: 6 | CALORIES PER SERVING: 225KCAL | TOTAL COOKING TIME: 30 MINS

INGREDIENTS

1   lb lean beef stew meat, cubed into bite sized pieces

1   tbsp olive oil

1   onion, chopped

2   carrots, peeled and diced

2   celery stalks, diced

3   cloves garlic, minced

4   cups low-sodium beef broth

3   cups water

3   potatoes, peeled and diced

1   cup green beans, trimmed and cut into bite-sized pieces

1   tsp dried thyme

1   tsp dried rosemary

1   bay leaf

Salt and pepper to taste

Chopped fresh parsley for garnish

METHOD

1. In a large pot, heat the olive oil over medium heat. Add the cubed beef and brown it on all sides. Remove the beef from the pot and set it aside.

2. In the same pot, add the chopped onion, diced carrots, and diced celery. Sauté for about 5 minutes, or until the vegetables start to soften.

3. Add the minced garlic and sauté for an additional 1 minute until fragrant.

4. Return the browned beef to the pot. Pour in the low-sodium beef broth and water. Stir to combine.

5. Add the diced potatoes, green beans, dried thyme, dried rosemary, and bay leaf. Season with salt and pepper to taste.

6. Bring the soup to a boil, then reduce the heat to low. Cover the pot and let the soup simmer for about 25-30 minutes, or until the beef is tender and the vegetables are cooked.

7. Once the soup is ready, remove the bay leaf and discard it.

8. Serve hot, garnished with chopped fresh parsley for added flavor and freshness.

PORK

SOUP

RECIPES

PORK NOODLE SOUP

SERVINGS: 4-6 | CALORIES PER SERVING: 225KCAL | TOTAL COOKING TIME: 40 MINS

INGREDIENTS

For the Broth:

8 cups low-sodium chicken or vegetable broth

1 onion, peeled and halved

3 cloves garlic, crushed

1-inch piece of ginger, sliced

1 star anise

1 cinnamon stick

2 cloves

1 tsp coriander seeds (optional)

Salt and pepper to taste

For the Soup:

8 oz lean pork tenderloin, thinly sliced

4 oz rice noodles, soaked and cooked according to package instructions

1 cup baby bok choy, chopped

1 carrot, julienned

1 red bell pepper, thinly sliced

1 green chilli, sliced

Fresh cilantro leaves, for garnish

Lime wedges, for serving

METHOD

1. In a large pot, combine the broth, onion, garlic, ginger, star anise, cinnamon stick, cloves, and coriander seeds (if using). Bring to a boil, then reduce the heat to a simmer. Let the broth simmer for about 20-30 minutes to infuse the flavors. Season with salt and pepper to taste.

2. While the broth is simmering, prepare the rice noodles according to the package instructions. Drain and set aside.

3. Remove the aromatics (onion, garlic, ginger, star anise, cinnamon stick, cloves) from the broth using a slotted spoon or strainer.

4. Add the sliced pork tenderloin to the broth and cook for a few minutes until the pork is cooked through and tender. Remove the pork slices from the broth and set aside.

5. In the same pot, add the chopped baby bok choy, julienned carrot, and sliced red bell pepper. Let the vegetables cook for a few minutes until they are slightly tender.

6. To assemble the soup, divide the cooked rice noodles among serving bowls. Top with the cooked pork slices and the cooked vegetables.

7. Ladle the hot broth over the noodles, pork, and vegetables. The hot broth will help heat the other ingredients.

8. Garnish the soup with sliced green chillies and fresh cilantro leaves.

9. Serve hot with lime wedges on the side for squeezing over the soup before eating.

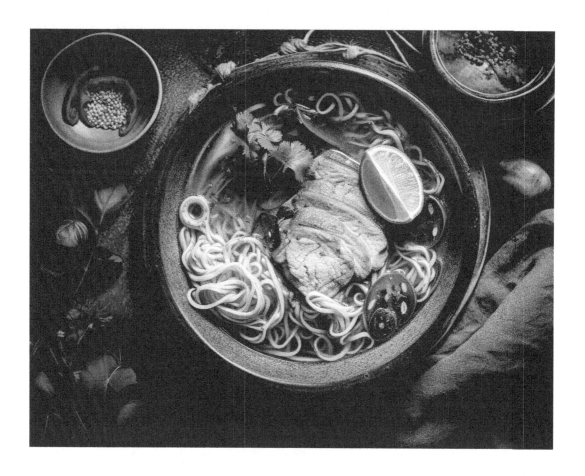

Root vegetables like carrots and potatoes add natural sweetness and body.

Texture Variety: Include ingredients with different textures for a more interesting mouthfeel.

Don't Overcook: Vegetables should be tender but not mushy.
Taste as you go.

SPICY PORK AND VEGETABLE SOUP

SERVINGS: 4-6 | CALORIES PER SERVING: 250KCAL | TOTAL COOKING TIME: 35 MINS

INGREDIENTS

1   tbsp olive oil
1   onion, chopped
3   cloves garlic, minced
1   tsp ginger, minced
1   lb (450g) lean ground pork
4   cups low-sodium chicken
    or vegetable broth
1   cup water
2   carrots, peeled and sliced
1   bell pepper
    (any color), chopped
1   zucchini, sliced
1   cup broccoli florets
1   tsp cumin
1   tsp paprika
½   tsp cayenne pepper
    (adjust to taste)
    Salt and pepper to taste
    Fresh cilantro or parsley,
    chopped (for garnish)
    Lime wedges (for serving)

METHOD

1. In a large soup pot, heat the olive oil over medium heat. Add the chopped onion, minced garlic, and minced ginger. Sauté for a few minutes until the onion is translucent and fragrant.

2. Add the lean ground pork to the pot. Break it apart with a wooden spoon and cook until it's browned and cooked through.

3. Stir in the cumin, paprika, and cayenne pepper. These spices will add a nice depth of flavor and a bit of heat to the soup. Adjust the amount of cayenne pepper based on your preference for spiciness.

4. Pour in the low-sodium chicken or vegetable broth and water. Bring the mixture to a simmer.

5. Add the sliced carrots, chopped bell pepper, zucchini, and broccoli florets to the pot. These vegetables will add vitamins, nutrients, and vibrant colors to the soup.

6. Let the soup simmer for about 15-20 minutes, or until the vegetables are tender but still slightly crisp.

7. Season the soup with salt and pepper to taste. Remember that some broth might already contain sodium, so taste before adding too much salt.

8. Once the vegetables are cooked to your liking, remove the soup from the heat.

9. Ladle the soup into bowls. Garnish each bowl with chopped fresh cilantro or parsley.

10. Serve the soup hot with lime wedges on the side. Squeezing a bit of lime juice into the soup just before eating adds a zesty and refreshing flavor.

PORK AND BEAN SOUP

SERVINGS: 4-6 | CALORIES PER SERVING: 225KCAL | TOTAL COOKING TIME: 45 MINS

INGREDIENTS

1 tbsp olive oil

1 lb (450g) lean pork loin, cubed

1 onion, chopped

2 carrots, peeled and diced

2 celery stalks, diced

3 cloves garlic, minced

1 can (14 oz/400g) low-sodium white beans, drained and rinsed

4 cups low-sodium chicken or vegetable broth

1 tsp dried thyme

1 tsp dried oregano

1 bay leaf

Salt and pepper to taste

2 cups fresh spinach or kale, chopped

Fresh parsley, chopped (for garnish)

METHOD

1. In a large pot, heat the olive oil over medium heat. Add the cubed pork and cook until browned on all sides. Remove the pork from the pot and set aside.

2. In the same pot, add the chopped onion, carrots, and celery. Sauté for a few minutes until the vegetables begin to soften.

3. Add the minced garlic, dried thyme, and dried oregano. Sauté for another minute until fragrant.

4. Return the cooked pork to the pot. Add the drained white beans and pour in the chicken or vegetable broth.

5. Add the bay leaf, and season with a pinch of salt and pepper. Stir to combine.

6. Bring the soup to a boil, then reduce the heat to low. Cover the pot and let the soup simmer for about 20-25 minutes, allowing the flavors to blend together.

7. About 5 minutes before serving, stir in the chopped spinach or kale. Let it wilt into the soup.

8. Taste and adjust the seasoning with more salt and pepper if needed. Remember to remove the bay leaf before serving.

9. Ladle into bowls, garnish with chopped fresh parsley, and serve hot.

PORK AND PUMPKIN SOUP

SERVINGS: 4-6　|　CALORIES PER SERVING: 200KCAL　|　TOTAL COOKING TIME: 45 MINS

INGREDIENTS

1　lb (450g) lean pork loin, cut into bite-sized pieces

2　cups diced pumpkin (you can also use butternut squash)

1　medium onion, chopped

2　cloves garlic, minced

1　carrot, peeled and chopped

1　tbsp olive oil

6　cups low-sodium chicken or vegetable broth

1　tsp dried thyme

½　tsp ground cumin

½　tsp ground cinnamon

　　Salt and pepper to taste

　　Fresh parsley or cilantro for garnish (optional)

METHOD

1.　Heat the olive oil in a large soup pot over a medium-high heat. Add the pork pieces and sear them until they are browned on all sides. This should take about 5 minutes. Remove the pork from the pot and set it aside.

2.　In the same pot, add the chopped onion, garlic, and carrot. Sauté for about 5 minutes or until the vegetables start to soften.

3.　Stir in the dried thyme, ground cumin, and ground cinnamon. Sauté for another minute to release their flavors.

4.　Return the seared pork to the pot, along with the diced pumpkin.

5.　Pour in the low-sodium chicken or vegetable broth. Bring the mixture to a boil, then reduce the heat to low. Cover and simmer for about 20-25 minutes or until the pork is cooked through, and the pumpkin is tender.

6.　Use an immersion blender or a regular blender to purée the soup until smooth. Be careful when blending hot liquids. If using a regular blender, allow the soup to cool slightly before blending in batches and then reheat it.

7.　Season the soup with salt and pepper to taste. Adjust the seasoning as needed. Ladle the soup into bowls and garnish with fresh parsley or cilantro, if desired.

8.　Serve the hot soup, accompanied by some whole-grain bread or a side salad for a complete meal.

PORK AND MUSHROOM SOUP

SERVINGS: 4-6　|　CALORIES PER SERVING: 200KCAL　|　TOTAL COOKING TIME: 35 MINS

INGREDIENTS

1   lb (450g) lean pork loin, thinly sliced

8   oz (225g) mushrooms, sliced

1   onion, chopped

2   carrots, peeled and sliced

4   cups low-sodium chicken or vegetable broth

4   cups water

2   cloves garlic, minced

1   tsp fresh ginger, grated

1   tsp olive oil

1   tsp soy sauce (low sodium)

1   tsp dried thyme

Salt and pepper to taste

Fresh parsley, chopped (for garnish)

METHOD

1. In a large pot, heat the olive oil over medium heat. Add the chopped onion and sauté for 2-3 minutes until translucent.

2. Add the minced garlic and grated ginger to the pot. Sauté for another minute until fragrant.

3. Add the sliced pork to the pot and cook until it's no longer pink (about 3-4 minutes).

4. Pour in the low-sodium chicken or vegetable broth and water. Stir in the sliced carrots and dried thyme. Bring the soup to a gentle boil, then reduce the heat to low. Cover the pot and let it simmer for about 15-20 minutes, allowing the flavors to blend.

5. Add the sliced mushrooms to the pot and let the soup simmer for an additional 5-7 minutes until the mushrooms are tender.

6. Season the soup with soy sauce, salt, and pepper to taste. Adjust the seasoning according to your preference.

7. Once the soup is fully cooked and the flavors have developed, remove it from the heat.

8. Ladle the pork and mushroom soup into serving bowls. Garnish each bowl with a sprinkling of freshly chopped parsley.

9. Serve the soup hot and enjoy its comforting and nourishing flavors.

PORK AND LENTIL SOUP WITH CURRY

SERVINGS: 4-6 | CALORIES PER SERVING: 225KCAL | TOTAL COOKING TIME: 50 MINS

INGREDIENTS

1   lb (450g) lean pork loin, trimmed of fat and cubed

1   cup dried green or brown lentils, rinsed and drained

1   onion, finely chopped

2   cloves garlic, minced

1   carrot, peeled and diced

1   celery stalk, diced

1   red bell pepper, diced

1   tbsp curry powder (adjust to taste)

1   tsp ground cumin

1   tsp ground coriander

½   tsp ground turmeric

6   cups low-sodium chicken or vegetable broth

2   bay leaves
    Salt and black pepper to taste

2   tbsp olive oil
    Fresh cilantro leaves for garnish (optional)

METHOD

1. In a large soup pot, heat the olive oil over medium-high heat. Add the cubed pork and sear until it's browned on all sides. Remove the pork from the pot and set it aside.

2. In the same pot, add the chopped onion, garlic, carrot, celery, and red bell pepper. Sauté for about 5 minutes or until the vegetables begin to soften.

3. Stir in the curry powder, cumin, coriander, and turmeric. Sauté for another minute to toast the spices, releasing their flavors and aromas.

4. Return the seared pork to the pot, along with the rinsed lentils. Stir everything together.

5. Add the chicken or vegetable broth and bay leaves to the pot. Bring the mixture to a boil.

6. Reduce the heat to low, cover the pot, and let the soup simmer for about 25-30 minutes or until the lentils and pork are tender.

7. Season the soup with salt and black pepper to taste. Remember that the broth might already contain some salt, so adjust accordingly.

8. Remove the bay leaves. Ladle the hot soup into bowls. Garnish with fresh cilantro leaves if desired.

This curried soup is a hearty and nutritious meal in a bowl. The lentils provide fiber and protein, while the lean pork adds a satisfying meatiness. The aromatic spices infuse the soup with rich flavors, making it a comforting choice for a cold winter's day.

PORK AND POTATO SOUP

SERVINGS: 4-6 | CALORIES PER SERVING: 215KCAL | TOTAL COOKING TIME: 50 MINS

INGREDIENTS

- 1 tbsp olive oil
- 1 onion, chopped
- 2 cloves garlic, minced
- 1 lb (450g) lean pork loin, trimmed and cubed
- 3 cups low-sodium chicken or vegetable broth
- 3 cups water
- 2 medium potatoes, peeled and diced
- 2 carrots, peeled and sliced
- 1 tsp dried thyme
- 1 tsp dried rosemary
- Salt and pepper to taste
- 2 cups chopped kale or spinach
- Fresh parsley, chopped (for garnish)

METHOD

1. In a large pot, heat the olive oil over medium heat. Add the chopped onion and sauté until translucent, about 3-4 minutes.

2. Add the minced garlic and cubed pork to the pot. Cook until the pork is browned on all sides.

3. Pour in the chicken or vegetable broth and water. Bring the mixture to a boil, then reduce the heat to low and cover the pot. Let the broth simmer for about 20 minutes to allow the flavors to blend.

4. Add the diced potatoes and sliced carrots to the pot. Stir in the dried thyme and rosemary. Season with salt and pepper to taste.

5. Cover the pot again and let the soup simmer for an additional 15-20 minutes, or until the potatoes are tender.

6. About 5 minutes before serving, stir in the chopped kale or spinach. Allow the greens to wilt slightly in the hot soup.

7. Taste the soup and adjust the seasoning if needed. If you prefer a thicker soup, you can use a potato masher to gently mash some of the potatoes and vegetables or you can leave as rustic.

8. Ladle into bowls. Garnish each bowl with chopped fresh parsley and enjoy!

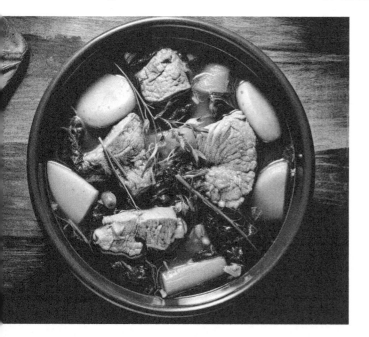

PORK AND MISO RAMEN SOUP

SERVINGS: 4-6 | CALORIES PER SERVING: 350KCAL | TOTAL COOKING TIME: 35 MINS

INGREDIENTS

1 lb (450g) pork loin or pork belly, thinly sliced

8 cups low-sodium chicken or pork broth

4 cloves garlic, minced

1-inch piece (2.5 cm) of ginger, sliced

2 tbsp miso paste (white or red, depending on your preference)

2 tbsp soy sauce (or tamari for a gluten-free option)

1 tbsp vegetable oil

1 onion, thinly sliced

2-3 green onions, chopped

2-3 boiled eggs, halved (optional)

1-2 cups fresh spinach or baby bok choy, chopped

8-10 ounces (284g) ramen noodles (use whole wheat or gluten-free noodles for a healthier option)

Salt and pepper to taste

METHOD

1. In a large pot, heat the vegetable oil over a medium-high heat. Add the minced garlic, ginger slices, and sliced onion. Sauté for a few minutes until fragrant and the onion becomes translucent.

2. Add the miso paste to the pot and stir well to combine with the other ingredients. Cook for an additional 2-3 minutes.

3. Pour in the chicken or pork broth and soy sauce (or tamari). Stir to combine all the ingredients.

4. Bring the broth to a simmer and let it cook for about 15-20 minutes, allowing the flavors to blend together. Season with salt and pepper to taste.

5. While the broth simmers, cook the ramen noodles according to the package instructions. Drain and set aside.

6. Heat a separate skillet over medium-high heat. Add a little oil if needed. Sear the thinly sliced pork until it's cooked through and slightly caramelized on the edges, about 2-3 minutes per side. Remove from heat.

7. Divide the cooked ramen noodles among serving bowls. Ladle the hot miso broth over the noodles.

8. Arrange the cooked pork slices, boiled eggs (if using), chopped spinach or baby bok choy, and green onions on top of the noodles and serve.

You can individualize this ramen with additional toppings like sliced mushrooms, bamboo shoots, bean sprouts, soft-boiled eggs, or seaweed.

PORK AND SWEET POTATO CHOWDER

SERVINGS: 4-6　|　CALORIES PER SERVING: 275KCAL　|　TOTAL COOKING TIME: 45 MINS

INGREDIENTS

- 1　lb (450g) lean pork tenderloin, cut into small cubes
- 2　medium sweet potatoes, peeled and diced
- 1　onion, chopped
- 2　cloves garlic, minced
- 2　carrots, peeled and chopped
- 4　cups low-sodium chicken broth
- 1　cup low-fat milk or unsweetened almond or coconut milk
- 1　tsp dried thyme
- ½　tsp smoked paprika
- Salt and black pepper to taste
- 2　tbsp olive oil
- Fresh parsley or chives for garnish (optional)

This Pork and Sweet Potato Chowder is not only delicious, but also a great source of lean protein and essential vitamins from the sweet potatoes.

METHOD

1. In a large soup pot, heat 1 tbsp of olive oil over a medium-high heat. Add the cubed pork and cook until browned on all sides. Remove the pork from the pot and set it aside.

2. In the same pot, add the remaining olive oil. Add the chopped onion, garlic, and carrots. Sauté for about 5 minutes until the vegetables begin to soften.

3. Stir in the diced sweet potatoes and continue to cook for another 5 minutes, allowing the sweet potatoes to slightly brown.

4. Return the seared pork to the pot. Add the dried thyme, smoked paprika, salt, and black pepper. Pour in the chicken broth and bring the mixture to a boil.

5. Reduce the heat to low, cover, and let the chowder simmer for about 20-25 minutes or until the sweet potatoes are tender and the pork is cooked through.

6. If you prefer a smoother chowder, use an immersion blender to blend some of the soup until you reach your desired consistency. Alternatively, you can use a potato masher to mash some of the sweet potatoes and thicken the chowder.

7. Stir in the low-fat milk or almond milk to add creaminess to the chowder. Heat the soup for an additional 5 minutes without boiling, just until warmed through.

8. Taste the chowder and adjust the seasoning with more salt and pepper if needed.

9. Ladle into bowls and garnish with fresh parsley or chives if desired.

PORK AND BEET BORSCHT

SERVINGS: 4-6 | CALORIES PER SERVING: 450KCAL | TOTAL COOKING TIME: 50 MINS

INGREDIENTS

For the Soup:

1 lb (450g) boneless pork loin or pork shoulder, cut into small cubes

2 tbsp olive oil

1 large onion, finely chopped

2 cloves garlic, minced

4 medium beets (beetroot), peeled and grated

3 carrots, peeled and grated

3 medium potatoes, peeled and diced

1 can (14 oz/400g) diced tomatoes

8 cups beef or vegetable broth (homemade or low-sodium store-bought)

2 bay leaves

1 tsp dried thyme

   Salt and pepper to taste

2 tbsp red wine vinegar (adjust to taste)

For the Garnish:

   Fat-free Greek yogurt or sour cream (for serving)

   Fresh parsley, chopped (for garnish)

METHOD

1. In a large soup pot, heat the olive oil over a medium-high heat. Add the pork cubes and brown them on all sides. Remove the pork from the pot and set it aside.

2. In the same pot, add the chopped onion and garlic. Sauté for about 5 minutes until the onions are translucent and fragrant.

3. Stir in the grated beets, grated carrots, and diced potatoes. Cook for another 5-7 minutes, allowing the vegetables to soften slightly.

4. Return the browned pork to the pot. Add the diced tomatoes (with their juice) and stir to combine.

5. Pour in the beef or vegetable broth and add the bay leaves and dried thyme. Season with salt and pepper to taste. Bring the mixture to a boil, then reduce the heat to low, cover, and simmer for about 30 minutes or until the pork is tender and the vegetables are cooked through.

6. Taste the soup and adjust the salt and pepper as needed. If you prefer a slightly tangy flavor, add the red wine vinegar a tbsp at a time, adjusting to your taste.

7. Ladle the hot borscht into bowls. Top each serving with a dollop of Greek yogurt or sour cream and a sprinkle of fresh dill or parsley.

8. Serve hot and enjoy the hearty and comforting flavors!

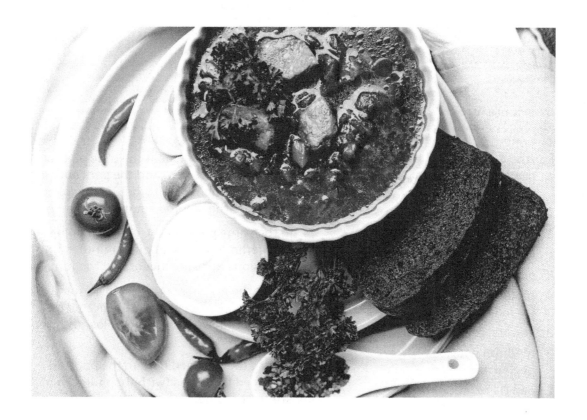

This Pork and Beet Borscht is not only delicious but also packed with vitamins and minerals from the beets, carrots, and pork. The touch of yogurt or sour cream on the side adds creaminess, and the fresh herbs provide a burst of freshness.

PORK AND TURMERIC SOUP

SERVINGS: 4-6 | CALORIES PER SERVING: 175KCAL | TOTAL COOKING TIME: 30 MINS

INGREDIENTS

1   lb (450g) lean pork
    loin, thinly sliced

1   small onion, finely chopped

2   cloves garlic, minced

1-inch (2.5cm) piece of
    fresh ginger, minced

2   carrots, peeled and julienned

1   cup spinach leaves, chopped

1   cup green beans, chopped

1   tsp ground turmeric

½   tsp ground cumin

½   tsp ground coriander

6   cups low-sodium
    chicken broth

1   tbsp olive oil
    Salt and pepper to taste
    Fresh cilantro or parsley
    for garnish (optional)

METHOD

1. Heat the olive oil in a large soup pot over a medium heat.

2. Add the chopped onion and sauté for about 3-4 minutes until it becomes translucent.

3. Stir in the minced garlic and ginger and cook for another minute until fragrant.

4. Add the sliced pork to the pot and cook for 3-4 minutes, or until the pork is lightly browned.

5. Sprinkle the ground turmeric, cumin, and coriander over the pork and stir well to coat the meat with the spices.

6. Pour in the chicken broth and bring the soup to a simmer. Cook for about 10 minutes, allowing the flavors to infuse.

7. Add the julienned carrots and chopped green beans to the pot. Simmer for an additional 5-7 minutes, or until the vegetables are tender but still crisp.

8. Stir in the chopped spinach and cook for another 2 minutes until the spinach wilts.

9. Taste the soup and season with salt and pepper as needed.

10. Ladle the hot soup into serving bowls and garnish with fresh cilantro or parsley if desired.

This soup is not only a flavorful and hearty meal but also packed with the anti-inflammatory benefits of turmeric. Enjoy it as a wholesome lunch or dinner, and you can customize it with your own favorite vegetables or herbs.

PORK AND APPLE CIDER SOUP

SERVINGS: 4-6　|　CALORIES PER SERVING: 275KCAL　|　TOTAL COOKING TIME: 45 MINS

INGREDIENTS

1　lb (450g) lean pork loin, cut into bite-sized cubes

2　tbsp olive oil

1　onion, finely chopped

2　cloves garlic, minced

2　medium apples, peeled, cored, and chopped (use sweet varieties like Gala or Fuji)

2　cups low-sodium chicken broth

1　cup apple cider

½　cup water

1　tsp dried thyme

½　tsp ground cinnamon

　　Salt and pepper to taste

　　Fat-free Greek yogurt or sour cream for garnish (optional)

　　Fresh parsley, chopped, for garnish (optional)

METHOD

1. Heat 1 tbsp of olive oil in a large pot or Dutch oven over a medium-high heat. Add the cubed pork and sear until browned on all sides. Remove the pork from the pot and set it aside.

2. In the same pot, add the remaining 1 tbsp of olive oil. Add the chopped onion and garlic. Sauté for about 3-4 minutes, or until the onion is translucent and fragrant.

3. Stir in the chopped apples, dried thyme, ground cinnamon, salt, and pepper. Cook for another 2-3 minutes, allowing the apples to soften slightly and absorb the flavors.

4. Pour in the low-sodium chicken broth, apple cider, and water. Stir well to combine all the ingredients.

5. Return the seared pork to the pot. Bring the mixture to a boil, then reduce the heat to low, cover, and let it simmer for about 20-25 minutes, or until the pork is tender and the apples are soft.

6. You can choose to leave the soup chunky or blend it to a smoother consistency. If blending, use an immersion blender directly in the pot, or transfer the soup in batches to a blender and blend until smooth. Be cautious when blending hot liquids.

7. Taste the soup and adjust the seasoning with more salt and pepper if needed.

8. Ladle the hot soup into bowls. Garnish with a dollop of Greek yogurt or sour cream and a sprinkle of chopped fresh parsley, if desired and serve.

PORK AND SHITAKE MUSHROOM CONGEE

SERVINGS: 4 | CALORIES PER SERVING: 325KCAL | TOTAL COOKING TIME: 50 MINS

INGREDIENTS

1 cup jasmine rice
(or any long-grain rice)

6 cups water or low-
sodium chicken broth

1 cup lean pork, thinly sliced

1 cup shiitake
mushrooms, sliced

2 cloves garlic, minced

1-inch piece (2.5cm) of
fresh ginger, minced

2 green onions, chopped
(separate the white
and green parts)

1 tbsp vegetable oil

1 tbsp soy sauce (low sodium)

1 tsp sesame oil

Salt and white pepper to taste

Fresh cilantro leaves
for garnish (optional)

Sliced red chili pepper
for garnish (optional)

This recipe isn't strictly a soup,
but I thought I'd add it anyway
as you cook it in a similar way
to a traditional soup. Congee
is a comforting and nutritious
rice porridge that's popular in
many Asian cuisines, perfect for
breakfast, lunch, or dinner. It's
packed with protein, fiber, and
rich umami flavors from the
shiitake mushrooms.

METHOD

1. Start by rinsing the rice thoroughly under
cold running water until the water runs
clear. Drain well and set aside.

2. In a large pot or Dutch oven, heat the
vegetable oil over a medium heat. Add the
minced garlic, ginger, and the white parts
of the green onions. Sauté for about 2
minutes or until fragrant.

3. Add the thinly sliced pork to the pot and
cook until it turns white and is no longer
pink. This should take about 3-4 minutes.

4. Stir in the sliced shiitake mushrooms and
cook for another 2-3 minutes until they
begin to soften.

5. Pour in the rinsed rice and give it a good
stir to combine with the other ingredients.
Then, add the water or chicken broth.
Bring the mixture to a boil.

6. Reduce the heat to low, cover the pot,
and let the congee simmer gently. Stir
occasionally to prevent the rice from
sticking to the bottom. Simmer for about
40-45 minutes, or until the rice has broken
down, and the congee has thickened to
your desired consistency (it should look
like a creamy porridge). If it becomes too
thick, you can add a little more water or
broth.

7. Season the congee with low-sodium soy
sauce, sesame oil, salt, and white pepper.
Adjust the seasonings to your taste.

8. Ladle the hot congee into bowls. Garnish
with the green parts of the chopped green
onions, fresh cilantro leaves, and sliced
red chili pepper for some heat if desired.

PORK AND CARROT SOUP

SERVINGS: 4-5 | CALORIES PER SERVING: 235KCAL | TOTAL COOKING TIME: 40 MINS

INGREDIENTS

1 tbsp olive oil
1 lb (450g) lean pork loin, diced
2 large carrots, peeled and chopped
1 onion, chopped
2 cloves garlic, minced
4 cups low-sodium chicken or vegetable broth
1 cup water
1 cup celery, chopped
1 cup green beans, trimmed and chopped
1 tsp dried thyme
1 bay leaf
   Salt and pepper to taste

METHOD

1. In a large pot, heat the olive oil over medium heat. Add the diced pork and cook until browned on all sides. Remove the pork from the pot and set it aside.

2. In the same pot, add the chopped onion and cook until it becomes translucent, about 3-4 minutes. Add the minced garlic and cook for an additional 1 minute.

3. Return the browned pork to the pot. Add the chopped carrots, celery, and green beans. Stir to combine.

4. Pour in the low-sodium chicken or vegetable broth and water. Add the dried thyme and bay leaf. Season with salt and pepper to taste. Stir well.

5. Bring the soup to a boil, then reduce the heat to low. Cover the pot and let the soup simmer for about 20-25 minutes, or until the vegetables are tender and the flavors have blended.

6. Once the vegetables are cooked, taste the soup, and adjust the seasoning if needed.

7. Remove the bay leaf from the soup and discard it.

8. Serve the pork and carrot soup hot. You can garnish it with fresh chopped parsley or a sprinkle of grated Parmesan cheese if desired.

PORK AND COCONUT SOUP

SERVINGS: 4-6 | CALORIES PER SERVING: 250KCAL | TOTAL COOKING TIME: 45 MINS

INGREDIENTS

1 lb (450g) lean pork tenderloin, thinly sliced

1 tbsp coconut oil

1 onion, finely chopped

2 cloves garlic, minced

1 tbsp fresh ginger, minced

1 red bell pepper, thinly sliced

1 carrot, peeled and thinly sliced

4 cups low-sodium chicken or vegetable broth

1 can (14 oz/400g) light or half-fat coconut milk

1 tbsp fish sauce (or soy sauce for a vegetarian option)

1 tbsp lime juice

1 tsp red curry paste (adjust to taste)

1 cup snow peas, ends trimmed and halved

Fresh cilantro leaves, for garnish

Salt and pepper, to taste

METHOD

1. Heat coconut oil in a large pot over medium heat. Add the sliced pork and cook until browned. Remove the pork from the pot and set aside.

2. In the same pot, add chopped onion, minced garlic, and minced ginger. Sauté until fragrant and the onion is translucent.

3. Add the red bell pepper and carrot slices. Cook for a few minutes until the vegetables start to soften.

4. Stir in the red curry paste and cook for another minute, allowing the flavors to blend in with each other.

5. Pour in the chicken or vegetable broth and bring the mixture to a gentle simmer.

6. Put the cooked pork back into the pot along with the halved snow peas.

7. Pour in the light coconut milk and fish sauce (or soy sauce). Stir well to combine all the ingredients.

8. Let the soup simmer for about 10-15 minutes, allowing the flavors to develop and the vegetables to become tender.

9. Just before serving, stir in the lime juice. Taste the soup and adjust the seasoning with salt and pepper if needed.

10. Ladle into bowls and garnish with fresh cilantro leaves for added flavor and a pop of color.

CHICKEN SOUP RECIPES

CLASSIC CHICKEN NOODLE SOUP

SERVINGS: 6 | CALORIES PER SERVING: 200KCAL | TOTAL COOKING TIME: 40 MINS

INGREDIENTS

1   tbsp olive oil

1   onion, diced

2   carrots, peeled and sliced

2   celery stalks, sliced

3   cloves garlic, minced

8   cups low-sodium chicken broth

2   boneless, skinless chicken breasts

1   tsp dried thyme

1   tsp dried oregano

1   bay leaf
    Salt and pepper to taste

2   cups whole wheat egg noodles

1   cup frozen peas
    Fresh parsley, chopped (for garnish)

METHOD

1. Heat the olive oil in a large pot over medium heat. Add the diced onion, sliced carrots, and sliced celery. Sauté for about 5 minutes until the vegetables start to soften.

2. Add the minced garlic and sauté for an additional 1 minute until fragrant.

3. Pour in the chicken broth and add the boneless chicken breasts, dried thyme, dried oregano, bay leaf, salt, and pepper.

4. Bring the soup to a boil, then reduce the heat to low. Cover the pot and let the soup simmer for about 20-25 minutes, or until the chicken is cooked through and tender.

5. Remove the chicken breasts from the pot and shred them using two forks.

6. Return the shredded chicken to the pot. Add the whole wheat egg noodles and frozen peas. Continue to simmer for an additional 8-10 minutes, or until the noodles are cooked to your desired level of tenderness.

7. Taste and adjust the seasoning with additional salt and pepper if needed. Remember to remove the bay leaf before serving.

8. Ladle the soup into bowls, garnish with freshly chopped parsley and serve.

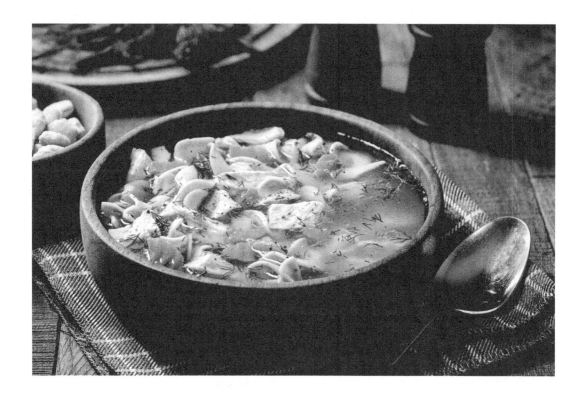

This healthier version of classic chicken noodle soup incorporates whole wheat noodles and plenty of vegetables for added nutrition. It's a comforting and nutritious meal that's perfect for warming up on chilly days or whenever you're in need of some comforting homemade soup.

CREAMY CHICKEN AND WILD RICE SOUP

· ·

SERVINGS: 4 | CALORIES PER SERVING: 250KCAL | TOTAL COOKING TIME: 50 MINS

INGREDIENTS

- 1 cup cooked wild rice
- 2 boneless, skinless chicken breasts, cooked and shredded
- 1 tbsp olive oil
- 1 onion, chopped
- 2 carrots, peeled and chopped
- 2 celery stalks, chopped
- 3 cloves garlic, minced
- 4 cups low-sodium chicken broth
- 1 tsp dried thyme
- 1 tsp dried rosemary
- ½ tsp dried sage
- 1 bay leaf
- 1 cup unsweetened almond milk (or milk of your choice)
- 2 tbsp whole wheat flour or alternative (like almond flour)
- Salt and pepper to taste
- Fresh parsley, chopped (for garnish)

METHOD

1. Cook the wild rice according to the package instructions. Set aside.

2. Cook the chicken breasts by grilling, baking, or poaching until fully cooked. Shred the cooked chicken using two forks, then set aside.

3. In a large pot, heat the olive oil over medium heat. Add the chopped onion, carrots, and celery. Sauté for about 5 minutes, or until the vegetables begin to soften.

4. Add the minced garlic, dried thyme, dried rosemary, dried sage, and bay leaf to the pot. Cook for an additional 1-2 minutes, until fragrant.

5. Sprinkle the whole wheat flour over the sautéed vegetables and stir to combine. Cook for 1-2 minutes to remove the raw taste of the flour.

6. Gradually pour in the chicken broth while stirring to avoid lumps. Add the almond milk and continue stirring until the mixture begins to thicken.

7. Add the shredded cooked chicken and cooked wild rice to the pot. Stir to combine all the ingredients.

8. Reduce the heat to low and let the soup simmer for about 15-20 minutes, allowing the flavors to blend together.

9. Taste the soup and add salt and pepper as needed. Remember that the chicken broth might already contain some salt, so adjust accordingly.

10. Ladle the creamy chicken and wild rice soup into bowls. Garnish with chopped fresh parsley for a burst of color and flavor.

This creamy chicken and wild rice soup is a delicious and nourishing option for a hearty meal. It's packed with protein, fiber, and vitamins from the vegetables and herbs. Plus, using almond milk and whole wheat flour creates a creamy texture without excessive amounts of dairy or refined flour.

Simmer Slowly: Slow simmering lets flavors blend. Avoid rapid boiling.

Use Natural Thickeners: Puree a portion of your soup for thickness instead of using flour or cornstarch.

Season Mindfully: Taste frequently and season with salt and pepper in small amounts, adjusting as needed.

Acid Balance: A splash of lemon juice or vinegar can brighten flavors.

LEMON CHICKEN ORZO SOUP

SERVINGS: 6 | CALORIES PER SERVING: 150KCAL | TOTAL COOKING TIME: 40 MINS

INGREDIENTS

1 tbsp olive oil

1 onion, diced

2 carrots, peeled and sliced

2 celery stalks, sliced

3 cloves garlic, minced

8 cups chicken broth
   (low sodium)

1 cup cooked chicken
   breast, shredded

½ cup uncooked orzo pasta

1 tsp dried thyme

1 bay leaf

   Zest and juice of 1 lemon

   Salt and pepper to taste

   Fresh parsley, chopped
   (for garnish)

METHOD

1. In a large pot, heat the olive oil over medium heat.

2. Add the diced onion, sliced carrots, and sliced celery. Sauté for about 5-7 minutes, or until the vegetables are slightly softened.

3. Add the minced garlic and sauté for another 1-2 minutes until fragrant.

4. Pour in the chicken broth and bring the mixture to a simmer.

5. Add the shredded cooked chicken to the pot and stir.

6. Add the uncooked orzo pasta, dried thyme, bay leaf, and lemon zest. Stir well.

7. Let the soup simmer for about 10-12 minutes, or until the orzo pasta is cooked al dente and the vegetables are tender.

8. Stir in the lemon juice. Taste and season with salt and pepper as needed. Adjust the amount of lemon juice to your preference.

9. Don't forget to remove the bay leaf from the soup before serving.

10. Serve and garnish each bowl with chopped fresh parsley.

You can customize this recipe by adding other vegetables, herbs, or spices that you like. Lemon adds a bright and zesty flavor to the soup, making it a perfect choice for a light and healthy meal.

MEXICAN CHICKEN TORTILLA SOUP

SERVINGS: 6 | CALORIES PER SERVING: 200KCAL | TOTAL COOKING TIME: 45 MINS

INGREDIENTS

For the Soup:

1 tbsp olive oil

1 onion, chopped

2 cloves garlic, minced

1 jalapeno pepper, seeds removed and finely chopped

1 red bell pepper, chopped

1 medium carrot, chopped

1 tsp ground cumin

1 tsp chili powder

½ tsp smoked paprika

4 cups low-sodium chicken or vegetable broth

1 can (14 ounces/400g) diced tomatoes

1 cup cooked and shredded chicken breast

1 can (14 ounces/400g) black beans, drained and rinsed

1 cup frozen corn kernels

Juice of 1 lime

Salt and pepper to taste

Chopped fresh cilantro for garnish

For Serving:

Baked corn tortilla strips or tortilla chips

Sliced avocado

Lime wedges

METHOD

1. Heat the olive oil in a large pot over medium heat. Add the chopped onion, garlic, jalapeno, red bell pepper, and carrot. Sauté for about 5-7 minutes, until the vegetables start to soften.

2. Stir in the ground cumin, chili powder, and smoked paprika. Cook for an additional 1-2 minutes to toast the spices.

3. Pour in the chicken or vegetable broth and diced tomatoes. Bring the mixture to a simmer.

4. Add the cooked and shredded chicken, black beans, and frozen corn. Allow the soup to simmer for about 15-20 minutes to allow the flavors to meld.

5. Squeeze in the juice of one lime and season the soup with salt and pepper to taste.

6. To serve, ladle the soup into bowls. Top each bowl with baked corn tortilla strips or tortilla chips, sliced avocado, and a squeeze of lime juice.

7. Garnish with chopped fresh cilantro for added flavor and serve.

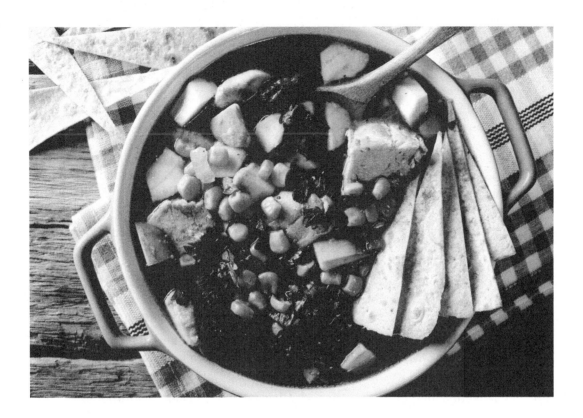

Note: You can adjust the level of spiciness by adding more or less jalapeno and chili powder, according to your taste preferences. Additionally, feel free to customize the toppings with grated cheese, fat-free Greek yogurt, or diced red onion if desired.

THAI COCONUT CHICKEN SOUP

SERVINGS: 4 | CALORIES PER SERVING: 350KCAL | TOTAL COOKING TIME: 45 MINS

INGREDIENTS

- 1 tbsp olive oil
- 1 lb (450g) boneless, skinless chicken breast or thigh, thinly sliced
- 4 cups chicken broth
- 1 can (14 oz/400g) coconut milk (full fat for creaminess)
- 2-3 kaffir lime leaves, torn into pieces
- 2 lemongrass stalks, cut into 2-inch (5cm) pieces and smashed
- 3-4 slices galangal or ginger
- 2-3 Thai red chilies, sliced (adjust to your spice preference)
- 1 cup sliced mushrooms (button or straw mushrooms)
- 1 medium tomato, cut into wedges
- 1 small onion, sliced
- 2-3 cloves garlic, minced
- 1 tbsp fish sauce (or soy sauce for a vegetarian version)
- 1 tbsp coconut sugar or brown sugar

Juice of 1-2 limes:

Fresh cilantro leaves for garnish

Salt to taste

METHOD

1. In a soup pot, heat a little oil over medium heat. Add the minced garlic and sliced onion. Sauté until the onion is translucent and fragrant.

2. Pour in the chicken broth and add the torn kaffir lime leaves, smashed lemongrass, galangal, or ginger slices, and sliced Thai red chilies. Bring the mixture to a gentle boil and let it simmer for about 5-10 minutes to infuse the flavors.

3. Add the sliced chicken to the pot and cook until the chicken is no longer pink.

4. Pour in the coconut milk and stir well. Allow the soup to gently simmer for another 5-7 minutes.

5. Add the sliced mushrooms and tomato wedges to the soup. Simmer until the mushrooms are tender and the tomatoes are softened.

6. Season the soup with fish sauce (or soy sauce for a vegetarian version), coconut sugar or brown sugar, and lime juice. Adjust the seasoning according to your taste preferences.

7. If you prefer a spicier soup, you can add a spoonful of Thai chili paste (nam prik pao) at this point.

8. Once everything is well combined and heated through, Discard the lemongrass, galangal or ginger slices, and kaffir lime leaves.

9. Ladle into serving bowls and garnish with fresh cilantro leaves.

Optional: Thai chili paste (nam prik pao) for extra flavor

10. Serve the soup hot as an appetizer or a light meal.

Also known as Tom Kha Gai. This soup is known for its rich and aromatic flavors, combining coconut milk, chicken, and fragrant Thai herbs. It's a comforting and satisfying dish that's perfect for any occasion.

Garnish Well: Fresh herbs, a dollop of yogurt, or a sprinkle of nuts can elevate your soup.

Experiment with Broth: Try different types of broth (chicken, vegetable, beef or fish) for unique flavor profiles.

Be Cautious with Spices: Some spices, like chili powder or red pepper flakes, intensify over time. Add them sparingly.

ITALIAN CHICKEN WEDDING SOUP

SERVINGS: 5 | CALORIES PER SERVING: 200KCAL | TOTAL COOKING TIME: 45 MINS

INGREDIENTS

For the Meatballs:

1   tbsp olive oil

(½ pound) 8 oz (225g) lean ground chicken or turkey

¼   cup whole wheat breadcrumbs

¼   cup grated Parmesan cheese

1   small egg

1   clove garlic, minced

½ tsp dried oregano

½ tsp dried basil

For the Soup:

1   tbsp olive oil

6   cups low-sodium chicken broth

1   cup small whole wheat pasta (such as orzo or small shells)

2   cups baby spinach, chopped

1   carrot, peeled and diced

1   celery stalk, diced

1   small onion, diced

2   cloves garlic, minced

½ tsp dried thyme

½ tsp dried oregano

Salt and pepper to taste

Fresh chopped parsley for garnish

Grated Parmesan cheese for garnish

METHOD

1. In a bowl, combine the ground chicken or turkey, breadcrumbs, grated Parmesan cheese, egg, minced garlic, dried oregano, dried basil, salt, and pepper.

2. Mix well until all ingredients are evenly combined, then shape the mixture into small meatballs, about 1 inch (2.5cm) in diameter.

3. In a large pot, heat a bit of olive oil over medium heat and add the meatballs and cook until browned on all sides. This step is for browning only; the meatballs will finish cooking in the soup. Remove the meatballs from the pot and set aside.

4. In the same pot, add a little more olive oil if needed, and sauté the diced onion, carrot, and celery until they begin to soften, about 3-4 minutes.

5. Add the minced garlic, dried thyme, dried oregano, salt, and pepper. Sauté for an additional 1-2 minutes until fragrant.

6. Pour in the low-sodium chicken broth and bring the soup to a gentle simmer.

7. Add the small whole wheat pasta and cook according to the package instructions.

8. Once the pasta is almost cooked, gently add the cooked meatballs back into the pot, then stir in the chopped baby spinach and let it wilt into the soup.

9. Ladle the soup into bowls and garnish with fresh chopped parsley and grated Parmesan.

CHICKEN AND CORN CHOWDER

SERVINGS: 5 | CALORIES PER SERVING: 235KCAL | TOTAL COOKING TIME: 35 MINS

INGREDIENTS

- 1 tbsp olive oil
- 1 onion, chopped
- 2 cloves garlic, minced
- 2 carrots, peeled and diced
- 1 red bell pepper, diced
- 1 tsp dried thyme
- 1 tsp dried oregano
- ½ tsp paprika
  Salt and pepper to taste
- 4 cups low-sodium chicken broth
- 2 cups cooked chicken breast, shredded
- 2 cups frozen corn kernels
- 1 cup low-fat milk or unsweetened almond milk
- 1 cup diced potatoes
- ½ cup plain fat-free Greek yogurt
  Chopped fresh parsley for garnish

METHOD

1. Heat the olive oil in a large pot or Dutch oven over medium heat.

2. Add the chopped onion and sauté for about 2-3 minutes, until translucent.

3. Stir in the minced garlic and cook for another 30 seconds, until fragrant.

4. Add the diced carrots, and red bell pepper to the pot. Cook for about 5-6 minutes, until the vegetables start to soften.

5. Sprinkle in the dried thyme, dried oregano, paprika, salt, and pepper. Stir to coat the vegetables with the spices.

6. Pour in the low-sodium chicken broth and bring the mixture to a simmer.

7. Add the cooked shredded chicken and frozen corn kernels to the pot. Let it simmer for about 10 minutes to allow the flavors to blend together.

8. In a separate small pot, boil the diced potatoes until they are fork tender. Drain and set aside.

9. Using an immersion blender or a regular blender, carefully blend a portion of the soup until creamy. This will help thicken the chowder without using heavy cream.

10. Return the blended soup to the pot and stir in the cooked diced potatoes.

11. Pour in the low-fat milk or unsweetened almond milk, and continue to cook for another 5 minutes, allowing the chowder to heat through.

12. Remove the pot from the heat and stir in the low-fat plain Greek yogurt. This will add creaminess and a touch of tanginess to the chowder.

13. Taste and adjust seasoning if needed.

14. Ladle the chowder into bowls, garnish with chopped fresh parsley and enjoy.

You can adjust this recipe by adding other vegetables like peas, green beans, bok choy, cabbage, or spinach for example.

Use Homemade Broth: If possible, make your own stock for richer, more nuanced flavors.

Mind the Simmer: A gentle simmer allows flavors to blend without scorching the bottom of the pot.

Leftovers: Soups often taste better the next day as flavors continue to blend. Store properly and reheat gently.

MOROCCAN SPICED CHICKEN SOUP

SERVINGS: 5 | CALORIES PER SERVING: 200KCAL | TOTAL COOKING TIME: 45 MINS

INGREDIENTS

For the Soup:

1   tbsp olive oil

1   onion, finely chopped

2   cloves garlic, minced

1   tsp ground cumin

1   tsp ground coriander

½   tsp ground turmeric

½   tsp ground cinnamon

¼   tsp ground ginger

¼   tsp cayenne pepper (adjust to taste)

½   tsp paprika

½   tsp saffron threads (optional)

1   large carrot, peeled and diced

1   red bell pepper, diced

1   zucchini, diced

1   cup diced tomatoes (canned or fresh)

6   cups chicken or vegetable broth

1   cup cooked shredded chicken breast

½   cup cooked chickpeas (canned or cooked from dried)

Salt and pepper to taste

Fresh cilantro or parsley, chopped (for garnish)

METHOD

1. In a large pot, heat the olive oil over medium heat. Add the chopped onion and sauté until translucent.

2. Add the minced garlic and all the ground spices (cumin, coriander, turmeric, cinnamon, ginger, cayenne pepper, and paprika). Stir well and cook for about 1-2 minutes until fragrant.

3. Add the diced carrot, red bell pepper, and zucchini to the pot. Sauté for a few minutes until the vegetables start to soften.

4. Pour in the diced tomatoes and saffron threads (if using). Stir to combine all the ingredients.

5. Pour in the chicken or vegetable broth and bring the soup to a simmer. Allow it to cook for about 15-20 minutes, or until the vegetables are tender.

6. Add the cooked shredded chicken and chickpeas to the soup. Simmer for an additional 10 minutes to heat the chicken and chickpeas through.

7. While the soup is simmering, prepare the couscous if using. Place the whole wheat couscous in a bowl and pour boiling water over it. Cover the bowl with a plate or lid and let it sit for about 5 minutes. Fluff the couscous with a fork and season with a pinch of salt.

8. Season the soup with salt and pepper to taste.

9. To serve, place a spoonful of cooked couscous in each bowl and ladle the Moroccan spiced chicken soup over it.

For the Couscous (optional):

½ cup whole wheat couscous

½ cup boiling water

　　Salt to taste

10. Garnish with chopped fresh cilantro or parsley.

11. Serve the soup hot with some whole grain bread or pita on the side if desired.

- -

Take out some of the soups liquid before blending and then ad back in gradually to reach your perfect consistency

- -

- -

Make vegetables the star of your soup for added nutrients and flavor.

- -

- -

Fresh herbs like parsley and cilantro add a burst of freshness without any extra calories.

- -

CHICKEN AND VEGETABLE SOUP

SERVINGS: 5 | CALORIES PER SERVING: 175KCAL | TOTAL COOKING TIME: 40 MINS

INGREDIENTS

1 tbsp olive oil

1 onion, chopped

2 cloves garlic, minced

2 carrots, peeled and diced

1 red bell pepper, diced

1 zucchini, diced

1 tsp dried thyme

1 tsp dried rosemary

1 tsp dried oregano

6 cups low-sodium chicken broth

2 boneless, skinless chicken breasts, cooked and shredded

1 cup green beans, trimmed and cut into bite-sized pieces

Salt and pepper, to taste

Fresh parsley, chopped (for garnish)

METHOD

1. Heat the olive oil in a large pot over medium heat. Add the chopped onion and cook until translucent, about 2-3 minutes.

2. Add the minced garlic, diced carrots, red bell pepper, and zucchini to the pot. Sauté for about 5 minutes, or until the vegetables start to soften.

3. Stir in the dried thyme, rosemary, and oregano, and cook for another minute until fragrant.

4. Pour in the chicken broth and bring the mixture to a simmer. Let it simmer for about 10-15 minutes, allowing the flavors to blend together.

5. Add the cooked and shredded chicken to the pot and stir to combine. Simmer for an additional 5 minutes.

6. Add the green beans to the soup and cook for about 5-7 minutes, or until the green beans are tender-crisp.

7. Season the soup with salt and pepper to taste. Adjust the seasoning according to your preferences.

8. Ladle into bowls and garnish with chopped fresh parsley for a burst of color and flavor.

CHICKEN AND DUMPLING SOUP

SERVINGS: 5 | CALORIES PER SERVING: 300KCAL | TOTAL COOKING TIME: 45 MINS

INGREDIENTS

For the Soup:

1   lb boneless, skinless chicken breasts or thighs, cubed
1   tbsp olive oil
1   onion, chopped
2   carrots, peeled and chopped
2   cloves garlic, minced
6   cups low-sodium chicken broth
1   cup frozen peas
1   tsp dried thyme
    Salt and pepper to taste
    Fresh parsley for garnish

For the Dumplings:

1   cup wholewheat flour
½   cup plain fat-free Greek yogurt
1   tsp baking powder
½   tsp salt
¼   cup milk (dairy or plant-based)

METHOD

1. In a large pot, heat the olive oil over a medium heat. Add the chopped onion and carrots, then sauté for about 5 minutes or until the vegetables begin to soften.

2. Add the minced garlic and sauté for another 1-2 minutes until fragrant.

3. Add the cubed chicken to the pot and cook until it's no longer pink on the outside.

4. Pour in the chicken broth and dried thyme. Season with salt and pepper to taste.

5. Bring the soup to a simmer and let it cook for about 15-20 minutes, allowing the flavors to blend and the chicken to cook right through.

6. Add the frozen peas during the last 5 minutes of cooking. Adjust the seasoning if needed.

7. While the soup is simmering, prepare the dumplings. In a mixing bowl, whisk together the whole wheat flour, baking powder, and salt.

8. Add the Greek yogurt and mix until crumbly.

9. Gradually add the milk, stirring until a soft dough forms. Be careful not to over-mix.

10. Once the soup is ready, drop spoons full of the dumpling dough onto the surface of the simmering soup.

11. Cover the pot with a lid and let the dumplings steam for about 10-12 minutes. They will puff up and become cooked in the steam from the soup.

12. Ladle the chicken and dumplings soup into bowls, making sure to get a good mix of vegetables, chicken, and dumplings in each serving.

13. Garnish with freshly chopped parsley for a burst of freshness.

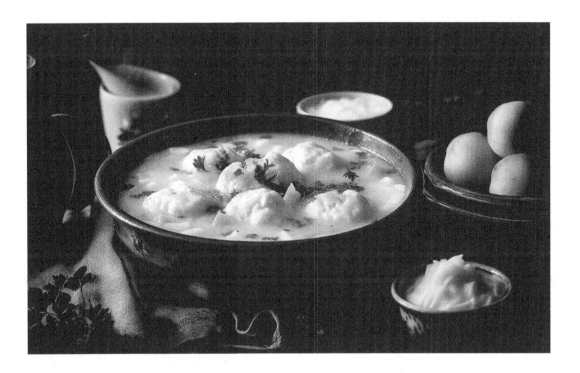

This version is designed to be healthier by using wholewheat flour for the dumplings and adding plenty of vegetables to the soup.

CHICKEN PHO

INGREDIENTS

For the Broth:

1 whole chicken (about 3-4 lbs/1.3-1.8 kg), preferably organic

1 large onion, peeled and halved

3-inch (7.6cm) piece of fresh ginger, sliced

4-5 cloves garlic, smashed

2 cinnamon sticks

3-4 star anise

6-8 whole cloves

1 tsp coriander seeds

1 tsp fennel seeds

8-10 cups water

For the Soup:

Rice noodles (enough for serving)

Cooked chicken meat (from the broth)

Fresh herbs: Thai basil, cilantro, mint

Bean sprouts

Lime wedges

Sriracha sauce or hoisin sauce (optional)

Sliced chili peppers (optional)

METHOD

1. Place the chicken, onion, ginger, and garlic in a large pot.

2. Dry roast the cinnamon sticks, star anise, cloves, coriander seeds, and fennel seeds in a separate pan until fragrant. Add these spices to the pot.

3. Cover the ingredients with water (about 8-10 cups) and bring to a boil. Skim off any foam that forms on the surface.

4. Reduce the heat to a gentle simmer and let the broth cook for about 1.5-2 hours, or until the chicken is tender and fully cooked.

5. Remove the chicken from the broth and let it cool slightly. Once cool enough to handle, shred the meat from the chicken and set it aside for serving.

6. Strain the broth through a fine mesh sieve into another pot. Discard any solids.

7. Taste the broth and adjust the flavor with salt and fish sauce if desired. The broth should be rich and aromatic.

8. Cook the rice noodles according to the package instructions. Rinse them with cold water after cooking to prevent them from sticking together.

9. In each serving bowl, place a portion of cooked rice noodles, then top with shredded chicken meat.

10. Ladle the hot broth over the noodles and chicken. The hot broth will help warm up the chicken and noodles.

Serve the Chicken Pho with a variety of fresh herbs, bean sprouts, lime wedges, and optional chili peppers. This is a Vietnamese noodle soup known for its flavorful broth and aromatic spices.

GREEK LEMON CHICKEN SOUP

SERVINGS: 4 | CALORIES PER SERVING: 160KCAL | TOTAL COOKING TIME: 40 MINS

INGREDIENTS

4 cups low-sodium chicken broth

2 cups cooked skinless chicken breast, shredded

½ cup uncooked orzo pasta or ¼ cup long grain rice

3 large eggs

Juice of 2-3 lemons (adjust to taste)

Zest of 1 lemon

Salt and pepper to taste

Fresh dill or parsley for garnish

Also known as Avgolemono Soup, this Greek soup is known for its delightful balance of flavors, with the bright tanginess of lemon and the richness of chicken. Its comforting flavors and creamy texture are achieved without using heavy cream. It is traditionally eaten at Easter to end the Lent fast.

METHOD

1. In a large pot, bring the chicken broth to a gentle simmer over medium heat.

2. Add the uncooked orzo pasta to the simmering broth. Cook according to the package instructions until the orzo is tender. This should take about 7-9 minutes.

3. Once the orzo is cooked, stir in the shredded chicken, and allow the mixture to heat through. Keep the soup on low heat to avoid boiling.

4. In a large mixing bowl, whisk the eggs until they are well beaten.

5. Gradually add the lemon juice to the beaten eggs, whisking constantly. This helps to temper the eggs and prevent them from curdling when added to the hot soup.

6. Slowly ladle about 1 cup of the hot broth from the pot into the egg-lemon mixture, whisking constantly. This further tempers the eggs.

7. Gradually pour the egg-lemon mixture back into the pot of soup, stirring gently to combine. Do not let the soup come to a boil at this point, as it can cause the eggs to curdle.

8. Add the lemon zest to the soup and stir to incorporate. Season with salt and pepper to taste. Adjust the amount of lemon juice if you prefer a more or less tangy flavor.

9. Continue to heat the soup over low heat, stirring gently, until it's heated through and has a slightly creamy consistency. Be careful not to let it boil.

10. Once the soup is warmed and the flavors are well combined, remove it from the heat.

11. Serve hot, garnished with fresh dill or parsley for a burst of flavor and color.

CHICKEN AND KALE SOUP

SERVINGS: 4 | CALORIES PER SERVING: 150KCAL | TOTAL COOKING TIME: 45 MINS

INGREDIENTS

1   tbsp olive oil

1   onion, chopped

2   carrots, peeled and chopped

3   cloves garlic, minced

1   tsp dried thyme

1   tsp dried rosemary

Salt and pepper to taste

4   cups low-sodium chicken broth

2   boneless, skinless chicken breasts, cooked and shredded

4   cups chopped kale, stems removed

1   cup diced tomatoes (canned or fresh)

Juice of 1 lemon

Fresh parsley, chopped (for garnish)

METHOD

1. Heat the olive oil in a large pot over medium heat. Add the chopped onion and carrots, then sauté for about 5 minutes, or until the vegetables begin to soften.

2. Add the minced garlic, dried thyme, dried rosemary, salt, and pepper. Cook for another 1-2 minutes until the garlic is fragrant.

3. Pour in the chicken broth and bring the mixture to a boil. Reduce the heat to low and let it simmer for about 10-15 minutes to allow the flavors to blend.

4. Add the cooked and shredded chicken to the pot. Stir to combine and let it simmer for an additional 5 minutes.

5. Add the chopped kale to the pot. Let the soup simmer for about 5-7 minutes, or until the kale is tender and wilted.

6. Stir in the diced tomatoes and lemon juice. Cook for another 2-3 minutes to heat the tomatoes through.

7. Taste the soup and adjust the seasoning with more salt and pepper if needed.

8. Ladle the soup into serving bowls. Garnish with chopped fresh parsley and serve.

This soup is not only delicious but also packed with nutrients from the kale and chicken. You can customize the recipe by adding other vegetables, beans, or whole grains for added texture and flavor.

CREAMY TOMATO BASIL CHICKEN SOUP

SERVINGS: 4 | CALORIES PER SERVING: 175KCAL | TOTAL COOKING TIME: 40 MINS

INGREDIENTS

1   tbsp olive oil

1   onion, chopped

2   cloves garlic, minced

2   carrots, peeled and diced

1   red bell pepper, diced

1   tsp dried basil

1   tsp dried oregano

½   tsp dried thyme

¼   tsp red pepper flakes
    (adjust to taste)

1   can (14 ounces/400g)
    crushed tomatoes

4   cups low-sodium chicken
    or vegetable broth

1   cup cooked and shredded
    chicken breast

½   cup light coconut milk
    or almond milk

    Salt and pepper, to taste

    Fresh basil leaves, for garnish

This creamy tomato basil chicken soup is rich, comforting, and packed with wholesome ingredients and can be served with wholegrain bread or a side salad for a complete and satisfying meal.

METHOD

1. Heat the olive oil in a large pot over medium heat. Add the chopped onion and sauté for 2-3 minutes until softened.

2. Add the minced garlic and sauté for another 30 seconds until fragrant.

3. Add the diced carrots, and red bell pepper to the pot. Sauté for about 5 minutes until the vegetables begin to soften.

4. Stir in the dried basil, dried oregano, dried thyme, and red pepper flakes. Cook for another minute to let the flavors meld.

5. Pour in the crushed tomatoes and chicken or vegetable broth. Bring the soup to a simmer.

6. Once the soup is simmering, add the shredded chicken. Let the soup simmer for 15-20 minutes to allow the flavors to develop and the vegetables to fully cook.

7. Use an immersion blender or transfer the soup to a regular blender (in batches) to purée the soup until smooth. If using a regular blender, return the puréed soup to the pot.

8. Stir in the light coconut milk or almond milk to create a creamy texture. If you prefer a thicker soup, you can add less milk or adjust based on your preference.

9. Season the soup with salt and pepper to taste. Keep in mind that canned tomatoes and broths can contain varying levels of sodium, so adjust accordingly.

10. Once the soup is heated through and seasoned to your liking, remove from heat.

11. Serve the soup in bowls, garnished with fresh basil leaves for an extra burst of flavor.

CHICKEN MULLIGATAWNY SOUP

SERVINGS: 6 | CALORIES PER SERVING: 300KCAL | TOTAL COOKING TIME: 45 MINS

INGREDIENTS

For the Soup:

1 tbsp coconut oil or olive oil

1 onion, finely chopped

2 carrots, peeled and diced

2 celery stalks, diced

1 red bell pepper, diced

2 garlic cloves, minced

1 tsp curry powder

½ tsp ground turmeric

½ tsp ground cumin

¼ tsp ground cinnamon

¼ tsp ground ginger

¼ tsp cayenne pepper
(adjust to taste)

1 cup red lentils, rinsed
and drained

1 cup cooked chicken
breast, shredded

6 cups low-sodium
chicken broth

1 can (14 ounces/400g) diced
tomatoes, undrained

Salt and pepper to taste

Juice of 1 lemon

Fresh cilantro or
parsley for garnish

Handful of roasted
cashews for garnish

METHOD

1. In a large soup pot, heat the coconut oil or olive oil over medium heat. Add the chopped onion, carrots, celery, and red bell pepper. Sauté for about 5-7 minutes until the vegetables are softened.

2. Add the minced garlic, curry powder, ground turmeric, ground cumin, ground cinnamon, ground ginger, and cayenne pepper. Sauté for an additional 1-2 minutes until fragrant.

3. Add the rinsed red lentils, shredded chicken, chicken broth, and diced tomatoes (with their juice) to the pot. Stir well to combine.

4. Bring the soup to a boil, then reduce the heat to low. Cover the pot and let the soup simmer for about 20-25 minutes until the lentils are tender and cooked through.

5. While the soup is simmering, prepare the coconut milk mixture. In a separate bowl, whisk together the coconut milk, curry powder, ground turmeric, and a pinch of salt. Set aside.

6. Once the lentils are cooked, carefully blend the soup using an immersion blender until you reach your desired consistency. You can leave it slightly chunky or blend it until it is smooth.

7. Return the blended soup to the pot and stir in the coconut milk mixture. Simmer the soup for an additional 5 minutes to heat through fully.

8. Season the soup with salt, pepper, and lemon juice to taste. Adjust the seasonings according to your preference.

For the Coconut Milk:

1 can (14 ounces/400g) coconut milk (full-fat or light)

½ tsp curry powder

½ tsp ground turmeric

   Salt to taste

9. Ladle into bowls and garnish with fresh cilantro or parsley.

10. Serve the soup hot with a side of wholegrain bread or naan, if desired.

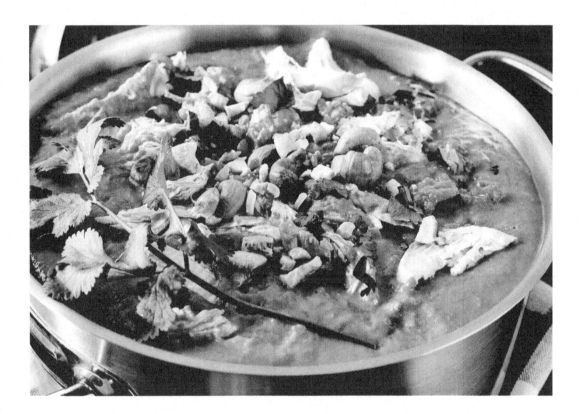

This Chicken Mulligatawny Soup is not only delicious but also packed with protein, fiber, and a blend of warming spices. It's a perfect filling and nutritious meal on its own. Mulligatawny soup originates from South India and its name comes from the Tamil words *milagu* and *tanni* meaning '*peppery water*'.

SEAFOOD SOUP RECIPES

CLASSIC CLAM CHOWDER

SERVINGS: 5 | CALORIES PER SERVING: 220KCAL | TOTAL COOKING TIME: 40 MINS

INGREDIENTS

2   cups fresh or frozen chopped clams (drained and juices reserved)

3   slices turkey bacon, chopped

1   onion, diced

2   celery stalks, diced

2   medium carrots, peeled and diced

2   cloves garlic, minced

3   cups low-sodium vegetable broth

2   cups low-fat milk (dairy or plant-based)

2   cups potatoes, peeled and diced

1   bay leaf

½   tsp dried thyme

¼   tsp dried oregano

¼   tsp black pepper

2   tbsp wholewheat flour

2   tbsp olive oil or unsalted butter

Chopped fresh parsley for garnish

Salt to taste

METHOD

1. In a large soup pot, heat olive oil over medium heat. Add the chopped turkey bacon and sauté until it starts to become crispy.

2. Add the diced onion, celery, and carrots to the pot. Sauté for about 5-7 minutes, or until the vegetables start to soften.

3. Stir in the minced garlic and cook for an additional 1-2 minutes until fragrant.

4. Sprinkle the wholewheat flour over the vegetables and stir well to coat. Cook for 1-2 minutes to remove the raw taste of the flour.

5. Slowly pour in the vegetable broth, stirring constantly to prevent lumps from forming. Add the reserved clam juice as well.

6. Add the diced potatoes, bay leaf, dried thyme, dried oregano, and black pepper to the pot. Bring the mixture to a simmer and let it cook for about 15-20 minutes, or until the potatoes are tender.

7. Once the potatoes are cooked, stir in the chopped clams and the milk. Simmer the chowder for an additional 5-7 minutes until the clams are heated through.

8. Taste the chowder and season with salt if needed. Remember that the clam juice and bacon might add some saltiness, so adjust accordingly.

9. Remove the bay leaf from the chowder and discard it.

10. Ladle the clam chowder into serving bowls. Garnish with chopped fresh parsley.

11. Serve with wholegrain crackers or a slice of wholewheat bread for a complete and satisfying meal.

SPICY SHRIMP AND CORN CHOWDER

SERVINGS: 4 | CALORIES PER SERVING: 250KCAL | TOTAL COOKING TIME: 35 MINS

INGREDIENTS

1   tbsp olive oil
1   medium onion, chopped
2   cloves garlic, minced
1   red bell pepper, chopped
1   jalapeño pepper,
    seeded and minced
    (adjust to taste)
2   cups frozen corn kernels
2   cups low-sodium
    vegetable broth
1   cup unsweetened
    almond milk (or any
    milk of your choice)
1   tsp smoked paprika
½   tsp cayenne pepper
    (adjust to taste)
1   tsp dried thyme
1   lb (450g) medium shrimp,
    peeled and deveined
    Salt and black pepper to taste
    Chopped fresh cilantro
    for garnish
    Lime wedges for serving

METHOD

1. In a large pot, heat the olive oil over medium heat. Add the chopped onion and cook until it becomes translucent, about 3-4 minutes.

2. Add the minced garlic, chopped red bell pepper, and minced jalapeño pepper to the pot. Sauté for another 2-3 minutes until the peppers are slightly softened.

3. Stir in the frozen corn kernels and cook for a few minutes until they begin to thaw.

4. Add the smoked paprika, cayenne pepper, and dried thyme to the pot. Stir to coat the vegetables with the spices.

5. Pour in the low-sodium vegetable broth and almond milk. Bring the mixture to a simmer and let it cook for about 10-15 minutes, allowing the flavors to blend together.

6. While the chowder is simmering, season the shrimp with a pinch of salt and black pepper.

7. Add the seasoned shrimp to the chowder and cook for about 4-5 minutes until the shrimp turn pink and opaque.

8. Taste the chowder and adjust the seasoning with more salt, black pepper, or cayenne pepper if desired.

9. Serve in bowls, garnished with chopped fresh cilantro and a lime wedge on the side.

This spicy chowder has a hint of sweetness from the corn and a refreshing, zing from the lime!

SEAFOOD THAI TOM YUM SOUP

SERVINGS: 4 | CALORIES PER SERVING: 250KCAL | TOTAL COOKING TIME: 30 MINS

INGREDIENTS

4   cups chicken or vegetable broth

1   stalk lemongrass, cut into 2-inch (5cm) pieces and lightly smashed

3-4 kaffir lime leaves, torn into pieces

3   slices galangal (or ginger if unavailable)

3-4 Thai bird's eye chilies, bruised (adjust to your spice preference)

1   small onion, sliced

2   cloves garlic, minced

7   oz (200g) mixed seafood (shrimp, squid, mussels, etc.)

7   oz (200g) mushrooms, sliced

1   tomato, cut into wedges

2   tbsp fish sauce

1   tbsp lime juice

1   tsp coconut sugar, stevia, or fruit sugar

Salt to taste

Fresh cilantro leaves for garnish

Optional:
Thai chili paste (Nam Prik Pao) for extra flavor

METHOD

1. In a pot, bring the chicken or vegetable broth to a simmer over a medium heat.

2. Add the lemongrass, kaffir lime leaves, galangal, Thai bird's eye chilies, onion, and garlic to the simmering broth. Let it cook for about 5-7 minutes to infuse the flavors into the broth.

3. Add the sliced mushrooms and tomato wedges to the pot. Continue simmering for another 3-4 minutes until the mushrooms are tender.

4. Add the mixed seafood to the pot and cook until they are just opaque and cooked through. This usually takes about 2-3 minutes, depending on the size of the seafood.

5. Season the soup with fish sauce, lime juice, and sugar. Adjust the seasonings according to your taste preferences. If you like it spicier, you can add more Thai bird's eye chilies or Thai chili paste (Nam Prik Pao).

6. Taste the soup and adjust the salt and other seasonings if needed.

7. Remove the pot from the heat and discard the lemongrass, kaffir lime leaves, galangal, and bruised chilies.

8. Ladle the soup into serving bowls and garnish with fresh cilantro leaves.

9. Serve the soup hot as a starter or a light main dish. You can enjoy it on its own or serve it with steamed jasmine rice.

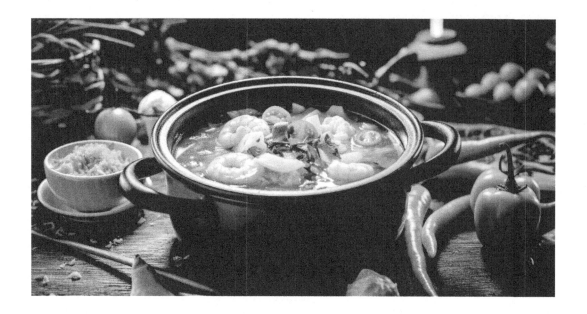

This recipe can also be adapted for vegetarian or vegan versions by using vegetable broth and omitting the seafood and using fresh vegetables instead.

SEAFOOD CIOPPINO

SERVINGS: 4 | CALORIES PER SERVING: 240KCAL | TOTAL COOKING TIME: 40 MINS

INGREDIENTS

- 1 tbsp olive oil
- 1 onion, finely chopped
- 2 cloves garlic, minced
- 1 bell pepper, diced
- 1 celery stalk, diced
- 1 carrot, peeled and diced
- 2 cans (14 oz/400g) crushed tomatoes
- 1 cup vegetable broth or fish stock
- ½ cup dry white wine (optional)
- 1 tsp dried oregano
- 1 tsp dried basil
- ½ tsp red pepper flakes (adjust to taste)
- Salt and black pepper to taste
- 1 bay leaf
- 8 oz (225g) firm white fish (such as cod or halibut), cut into chunks
- 8 oz (225g) shrimp, peeled and deveined
- 8 oz (225g) mussels or clams, scrubbed and debearded
- 4 oz (113g) calamari rings
- Fresh basil or parsley, chopped, for garnish

METHOD

1. In a large pot or Dutch oven, heat the olive oil over medium heat. Add the chopped onion and sauté until translucent, about 3-4 minutes.

2. Add the minced garlic, diced bell pepper, diced celery, and diced carrot. Sauté for another 3-4 minutes, until the vegetables start to soften.

3. Pour in the crushed tomatoes, vegetable broth or fish stock, and dry white wine (if using). Stir to combine.

4. Add the dried oregano, dried basil, red pepper flakes, salt, black pepper, and bay leaf. Stir to incorporate the seasonings.

5. Bring the mixture to a simmer and let it cook for about 15-20 minutes, allowing the flavors to blend together and the vegetables to become tender.

6. Once the base of the stew has simmered, add the chunks of firm white fish, shrimp, mussels or clams, and calamari rings. Gently add the seafood into the liquid.

7. Cover the pot and let the seafood cook for about 5-7 minutes, or until the shrimp turns pink and the mussels or clams open. Discard any mussels or clams that remain closed.

8. Taste and adjust the seasoning if needed. Remember that seafood will give a natural saltiness to the stew.

9. Once the seafood is cooked through, remove the pot from the heat and discard the bay leaf.

10. Ladle into serving bowls. Garnish with freshly chopped basil or parsley.

11. You can serve Cioppino with crusty wholegrain bread or a side of cooked pasta, if desired.

LOBSTER BISQUE

SERVINGS: 4 | CALORIES PER SERVING: 180KCAL | TOTAL COOKING TIME: 45 MINS

INGREDIENTS

- 2 lobster tails (about 8 oz/225g each), shells removed, and meat chopped into bite-sized pieces
- 1 small onion, chopped
- 2 cloves garlic, minced
- 1 carrot, peeled and chopped
- 1 small potato, peeled and chopped
- 2 cups low-sodium vegetable broth
- 1 cup reduced-fat milk or unsweetened almond, oat, or coconut milk
- ¼ cup plain fat-free Greek yogurt
- 1 tbsp olive oil
- 1 tbsp wholewheat flour
- ¼ tsp paprika
- ¼ tsp dried thyme
- Salt and black pepper to taste
- Fresh chives or parsley for garnish

METHOD

1. In a large pot, heat the olive oil over medium heat. Add the chopped onion, garlic, and carrot. Sauté for about 5 minutes, until the vegetables start to soften.

2. Sprinkle the whole wheat flour over the sautéed vegetables. Stir well to coat the vegetables with the flour.

3. Pour in the vegetable broth and add the chopped potato. Bring the mixture to a simmer and let it cook for about 15-20 minutes, or until the potato is tender.

4. Use an immersion blender or a regular blender to purée the soup until smooth. If using a regular blender, make sure to blend in batches and be cautious of hot liquid.

5. Return the puréed soup to the pot and stir in the paprika, dried thyme, salt, and black pepper.

6. Add the chopped lobster meat to the soup and let it simmer for an additional 5-7 minutes, until the lobster is cooked and tender.

7. Reduce the heat to low and stir in the reduced-fat milk or almond milk. Let the soup warm through but avoid boiling it.

8. Remove the pot from the heat and whisk in the Greek yogurt until the soup becomes creamy.

9. Taste and adjust the seasoning as needed and ladle into serving bowls. Garnish with fresh chives or parsley.

Enjoy this healthier version of lobster bisque that still captures the luxurious taste of the classic dish without the excessive calories and fat. Serve it with wholegrain bread or a side salad for a complete meal.

MEDITERRANEAN BOUILLABAISSE

SERVINGS: 4 | CALORIES PER SERVING: 325KCAL | TOTAL COOKING TIME: 45 MINS

INGREDIENTS

1   lb mixed fish fillets (such as cod, halibut, snapper), cut into bite-sized chunks
8-10 large shrimp, peeled and deveined
8-10 mussels, cleaned and debearded
1   onion, chopped
2   cloves garlic, minced
1   fennel bulb, thinly sliced
1   red bell pepper, chopped
1   can (14 oz/400g) diced tomatoes, with juice
2   cups vegetable broth or fish stock
½   cup dry white wine (optional)
¼   cup extra-virgin olive oil
1   tsp saffron threads
1   tsp dried thyme
1   tsp dried oregano
1   bay leaf
    Salt and pepper, to taste
    Fresh parsley, chopped, for garnish
    Slices of wholegrain baguette, for serving

This delicious French Provençal soup was first created in the port of Marseille by fishermen not wanting to waste any leftover scraps from their catch. The name comes from two French Occitan words *bothir* and *abaisser* meaning to *boil* and to *reduce heat.*

METHOD

1. In a large pot or Dutch oven, heat the olive oil over medium heat. Add the chopped onion, sliced fennel, and red bell pepper. Sauté for about 5-7 minutes, or until the vegetables are softened.

2. Add the minced garlic, dried thyme, dried oregano, and saffron threads to the pot. Sauté for an additional minute, allowing the spices to release their flavors.

3. Pour in the vegetable broth or fish stock and the diced tomatoes with their juice. If using, add the dry white wine as well. Stir to combine.

4. Add the bay leaf to the pot and season with salt and pepper to taste. Bring the mixture to a gentle simmer and cook for about 15-20 minutes, allowing the flavors to blend.

5. Carefully add the fish chunks and shrimp to the pot. Make sure they are submerged in the broth. Cover the pot and let the seafood cook for about 5-7 minutes, or until the fish is opaque and the shrimp are pink and curled.

6. Gently add the cleaned mussels to the pot, making sure they are distributed evenly. Cover the pot and cook for an additional 5-7 minutes, or until the mussels have opened.

7. Taste the broth and adjust the seasoning if needed. Discard any mussels that haven't opened.

8. To serve, ladle into bowls, making sure each bowl has a good variety of fish, shrimp, and mussels. Sprinkle with chopped fresh parsley for a burst of color and flavor.

SEAFOOD GUMBO

SERVINGS: 4 | CALORIES PER SERVING: 375KCAL | TOTAL COOKING TIME: 60 MINS

INGREDIENTS

For the Gumbo Base:

2 tbsp olive oil

1 onion, chopped

1 green bell pepper, chopped

2 celery stalks, chopped

3 cloves garlic, minced

2 tbsp wholewheat flour (or another flour of your choice)

1 tsp paprika

½ tsp dried thyme

½ tsp dried oregano

¼ tsp cayenne pepper (adjust to taste)

1 can (14 oz/400g) diced tomatoes (low sodium)

4 cups low-sodium seafood or vegetable broth

Salt and black pepper to taste

For the Seafood:

8 oz (225g) white fish fillets (such as cod or snapper), cut into bite-sized pieces

8 oz (225g) medium shrimp, peeled and deveined

8 oz (225g) bay scallops

1 tbsp Cajun seasoning (low sodium)

Juice of 1 lemon

METHOD

1. Heat the olive oil in a large pot or Dutch oven over medium heat. Add the chopped onion, green bell pepper, and celery. Sauté for about 5 minutes, or until the vegetables are softened.

2. Stir in the minced garlic and cook for an additional 1-2 minutes until fragrant.

3. Sprinkle the flour over the vegetables and stir to combine. Cook for 2-3 minutes, stirring occasionally, to cook off the raw flour taste.

4. Add the paprika, dried thyme, dried oregano, and cayenne pepper to the pot. Stir well to coat the vegetables and flour with the spices.

5. Pour in the diced tomatoes with their juice. Stir to combine.

6. Gradually add the seafood or vegetable broth, stirring continuously to prevent lumps from forming. Bring the mixture to a simmer.

7. Season the gumbo base with salt and black pepper to taste. Let the mixture simmer for about 15-20 minutes, allowing the flavors to blend.

8. While the gumbo base is simmering, prepare the seafood. In a bowl, toss the white fish, shrimp, and bay scallops with Cajun seasoning and lemon juice. Let them marinate briefly.

9. Gently add the marinated seafood to the simmering gumbo base. Cook for about 5-7 minutes, or until the seafood is cooked through and the shrimp turns pink.

For Serving:

Cooked brown rice or quinoa

Chopped fresh parsley
or green onions
(scallions) for garnish

10. Taste and adjust the seasoning if needed. If the gumbo is too thick, you can add a little more broth to achieve your desired consistency.

11. Serve over cooked brown rice or quinoa. Garnish with chopped fresh parsley or green onions.

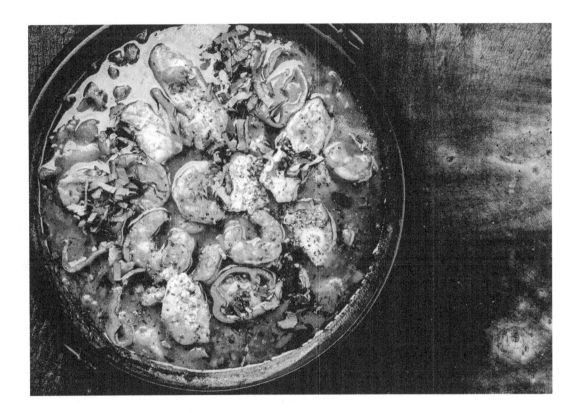

A Gumbo is such a hearty soup that it can also be described as a casserole too! It hails from the state of Louisiana in the United States. Its hallmark is that it always contains the 'holy trinity' of Cajun cooking - onions, celery, and bell peppers.

MEDITERRANEAN SEAFOOD SOUP

SERVINGS: 4 | CALORIES PER SERVING: 300KCAL | TOTAL COOKING TIME: 35 MINS

INGREDIENTS

2   tbsp olive oil

1   onion, finely chopped

2   cloves garlic, minced

1   red bell pepper, diced

1   yellow bell pepper, diced

1   fennel bulb, thinly sliced

1   tsp dried oregano

½ tsp red pepper flakes
    (adjust to taste)

1   can (14 oz/400g) diced
    tomatoes, with juice

4   cups seafood or fish broth

1   cup dry white wine (optional)

1   bay leaf
    Salt and black pepper to taste

1   lb (450g) mixed seafood
    (such as shrimp, mussels,
    clams, and firm white fish),
    cleaned and deveined

½ cup chopped fresh parsley
    Fresh lemon wedges,
    for serving

Also known as "Cioppino",
this hearty Italian soup is rich
in seafood and vegetables,
making it a perfect choice for
a healthy and hearty meal that
perfectly captures the flavors
of the sea. Cioppino became
popular in San Francisco in the
19th century where it was made
by Italian fishermen working
there.

METHOD

1. In a large pot or Dutch oven, heat the olive oil over medium heat. Add the chopped onion and sauté until translucent, about 3-4 minutes.

2. Add the minced garlic, diced red and yellow bell peppers, and sliced fennel. Cook for an additional 4-5 minutes, until the vegetables start to soften.

3. Stir in the dried oregano and red pepper flakes and cook for another minute until fragrant.

4. Add the diced tomatoes (with their juice), seafood or fish broth, dry white wine (if using), bay leaf, salt, and black pepper. Bring the mixture to a gentle simmer, then reduce the heat to low. Cover the pot and let the flavors blend for about 20-25 minutes.

5. Once the soup base has simmered and the flavors are well combined, carefully add the mixed seafood to the pot. Cook for about 5-7 minutes, or until the seafood is fully cooked. The shrimp should turn pink, mussels and clams should open, and the fish should be opaque and flaky.

6. Taste the soup and adjust the seasoning with more salt and pepper if needed.

7. Remove the pot from the heat and discard the bay leaf.

8. Serve in bowls, garnished with chopped fresh parsley and a squeeze of fresh lemon juice. The lemon juice adds a bright and refreshing flavor to the soup.

9. Serve the soup with crusty wholegrain bread or a side salad for a complete and satisfying meal.

KOREAN SPICY SEAFOOD SOUP

SERVINGS: 4 | CALORIES PER SERVING: 175KCAL | TOTAL COOKING TIME: 40 MINS

INGREDIENTS

½ cup medium-sized shrimp, peeled and deveined

½ cup squid rings (cleaned)

½ cup mussels or clams, cleaned

½ cup firm white fish fillets, cut into bite-sized pieces

4 cups seafood or vegetable broth

1 small onion, thinly sliced

2 cloves garlic, minced

1 small zucchini, thinly sliced

½ cup tofu, cubed

½ cup enoki mushrooms (or other mushrooms of choice)

2 green onions, chopped

2 tbsp Korean red pepper paste (gochujang)

1 tbsp Korean red pepper flakes (gochugaru)

1 tbsp soy sauce

1 tsp sesame oil

Salt and pepper to taste

1 tbsp vegetable oil

Fresh cilantro or parsley for garnish (optional)

Cooked rice for serving

METHOD

1. Heat the vegetable oil in a large pot over medium heat. Add the sliced onion and minced garlic. Sauté for a few minutes until the onion becomes translucent and fragrant.

2. Add the seafood (shrimp, squid, mussels or clams, and fish) to the pot. Cook for a couple of minutes until the seafood starts to turn opaque.

3. Add the seafood or vegetable broth to the pot. Bring the broth to a simmer and let the seafood cook for a few more minutes until fully cooked. Remove any shells that don't open.

4. Stir in the Korean red pepper paste (gochujang) and red pepper flakes (gochugaru). These will give the soup its signature spicy flavor. Adjust the amount to your spice preference.

5. Add the sliced zucchini, tofu, and mushrooms to the soup. Let the soup simmer for about 5-7 minutes until the vegetables are tender.

6. Season the soup with soy sauce, sesame oil, salt, and pepper. Taste and adjust the seasoning as needed.

7. Just before serving, sprinkle chopped green onions over the soup.

8. Ladle into bowls and garnish with fresh cilantro or parsley if desired.

9. Serve the soup hot with a side of cooked rice.

Known in Korea as "Haemul Jjigae," this spicy seafood soup is a comforting and hearty dish with a delightful balance of spiciness and umami flavors from the seafood and vegetables.

BRAZILIAN SEAFOOD MOQUECA

SERVINGS: 4 | CALORIES PER SERVING: 275KCAL | TOTAL COOKING TIME: 40 MINS

INGREDIENTS

For the Marinade:

1   lb mixed seafood
    (shrimp, fish, squid),
    cleaned and deveined
    Juice of 1 lime
    Salt and pepper to taste

For the Moqueca:

1   tbsp olive oil
1   onion, finely chopped
2   cloves garlic, minced
1   red bell pepper, sliced
1   green bell pepper, sliced
2   tomatoes, chopped
1   tbsp paprika
1   tsp ground cumin
1   tsp ground coriander
½   tsp red pepper flakes
    (adjust to taste)
1   can (14 oz/400g) coconut
    milk (half-fat or light)
½   cup fish or vegetable broth
    Salt and pepper to taste
    Chopped fresh cilantro
    or parsley for garnish
    Lime wedges for serving

METHOD

1. Start by marinating the seafood. In a bowl, combine the mixed seafood, lime juice, salt, and pepper. Toss to coat the seafood well with the marinade. Let it marinate for about 15-20 minutes while you prepare the other ingredients.

2. In a large pot or deep skillet, heat the olive oil over medium heat. Add the chopped onion and sauté until translucent.

3. Add the minced garlic and sliced bell peppers to the pot. Cook for a few minutes until the peppers start to soften.

4. Stir in the chopped tomatoes, paprika, ground cumin, ground coriander, and red pepper flakes. Cook for another 5 minutes, allowing the flavors to blend.

5. Pour in the coconut milk and fish or vegetable broth. Bring the mixture to a gentle simmer.

6. Carefully add the marinated seafood to the pot, along with any accumulated juices. Allow the seafood to cook in the simmering liquid for about 5-7 minutes, or until the shrimp turn pink and the fish is cooked through.

7. Season the moqueca with salt and pepper to taste. Adjust the seasoning and spiciness level according to your preference.

8. Once the seafood is cooked and the flavors have developed, remove the pot from the heat. Garnish the moqueca with chopped fresh cilantro or parsley.

9. Serve hot, with lime wedges on the side for squeezing over the dish. It's commonly enjoyed with steamed rice or crusty bread to soak up the delicious sauce.

MEXICAN SEAFOOD SOUP

SERVINGS: 5 | CALORIES PER SERVING: 225KCAL | TOTAL COOKING TIME: 40 MINS

INGREDIENTS

1 tbsp olive oil
1 onion, chopped
2 cloves garlic, minced
1 bell pepper, diced (any color)
2 tomatoes, diced
1 tsp ground cumin
1 tsp paprika
½ tsp dried oregano
¼ tsp cayenne pepper
   (adjust to taste)
6 cups fish or seafood broth
   (homemade or low sodium)
1 cup water
1 lb (450g) mixed seafood
   (shrimp, fish, mussels,
   clams, squid), cleaned
   and chopped
1 cup corn kernels (fresh,
   frozen, or canned)
1 zucchini, diced
   Juice of 1 lime
   Salt and black pepper to taste
   Fresh cilantro, chopped,
   for garnish
   Sliced avocado, for serving
   Lime wedges, for serving

Optional: hot sauce or chili
flakes for extra heat

"Caldo de Mariscos" as it is
known in Mexico is a flavorful
soup, packed with a variety
of seafood and aromatic
ingredients. This soup is often
called Caldo de Siete Mares –
'Seven Seas Soup' and is served
in all Mexican coastal regions...

METHOD

1. In a large pot, heat the olive oil over
   medium heat. Add the chopped onion and
   sauté until translucent.

2. Add the minced garlic and diced bell
   pepper to the pot. Sauté for a couple of
   minutes until the bell pepper starts to
   soften.

3. Stir in the diced tomatoes, ground cumin,
   paprika, dried oregano, and cayenne
   pepper. Cook for a few minutes until the
   tomatoes start to break down and release
   their juices.

4. Pour in the fish or seafood broth and water.
   Bring the soup to a simmer and let it cook
   gently for about 10-15 minutes to allow the
   flavors to blend.

5. Add the mixed seafood to the simmering
   soup. Cook for a few minutes until the
   seafood turns opaque and is cooked
   through. Be careful not to overcook the
   seafood, as it can become tough.

6. Add the corn kernels and diced zucchini to
   the pot. Let the soup simmer for another
   5-7 minutes until the zucchini is tender.

7. Squeeze in the juice of one lime and
   season the soup with salt and black
   pepper to taste. Adjust the seasoning and
   add extra cayenne pepper if you prefer a
   spicier soup.

8. Once the soup is ready, ladle it into serving
   bowls. Garnish with chopped cilantro and
   avocado slices.

9. Serve with lime wedges on the side for
   squeezing over the soup. If you enjoy extra
   heat, you can add hot sauce or chili flakes
   as well.

GREEK SEAFOOD SOUP

. . . .

SERVINGS: 4 | CALORIES PER SERVING: 250KCAL | TOTAL COOKING TIME: 40 MINS

INGREDIENTS

- 1 tbsp olive oil
- 1 onion, finely chopped
- 2 garlic cloves, minced
- 1 carrot, peeled and chopped
- 1 small fennel bulb, chopped
- 1 bay leaf
- 1 tsp dried oregano
- 1 tsp dried thyme
- 1 tsp dried dill
- 1 can (14 oz/400g) diced tomatoes
- 6 cups fish or seafood broth (homemade or store-bought)
- 1 cup water
- ½ cup dry white wine (optional)
- 1 potato, peeled and diced
- ½ lb (225g) firm white fish fillets (such as cod or haddock), cut into chunks
- ½ lb (225g) shrimp, peeled and deveined
- ½ lb (225g) mussels or clams, cleaned
- Salt and pepper to taste
- Fresh lemon juice, for serving
- Chopped fresh parsley, for garnish

METHOD

1. In a large pot, heat the olive oil over medium heat. Add the chopped onion, garlic, carrot, and fennel. Sauté for about 5 minutes, or until the vegetables start to soften.

2. Add the bay leaf, dried oregano, dried thyme, and dried dill to the pot. Sauté for another minute to release the flavors.

3. Pour in the diced tomatoes (with their juices) and cook for a few minutes to allow the flavors to blend.

4. Add the fish or seafood broth, water, and dry white wine (if using). Stir to combine.

5. Add the diced potato to the pot. Bring the soup to a gentle simmer and let it cook for about 15-20 minutes, or until the potato is tender.

6. Once the potato is cooked, add the chunks of white fish fillets, shrimp, and mussels or clams to the soup. Simmer for an additional 5-7 minutes, or until the seafood is cooked through. Discard any mussels or clams that do not open.

7. Season the soup with salt and pepper to taste. Remember that seafood broth can be naturally salty, so be cautious with the salt.

8. Remove the pot from the heat and discard the bay leaf.

9. Serve the soup in bowls. Squeeze a bit of fresh lemon juice over each serving for a burst of flavor and a sprinkling of chopped fresh parsley.

"Psarosoupa" as it is called in Greece is a traditional flavorful seafood soup that captures the essence of Mediterranean cuisine. Serve with extra lemon wedges to squeeze over the soup.

SPANISH SEAFOOD SOUP

SERVINGS: 4 | CALORIES PER SERVING: 300KCAL | TOTAL COOKING TIME: 35 MINS

INGREDIENTS

1   tbsp olive oil

1   onion, finely chopped

2   cloves garlic, minced

1   red bell pepper, diced

1   green bell pepper, diced

1   carrot, peeled and diced

1   tsp smoked paprika

½   tsp cayenne pepper
    (adjust to taste)

1   tsp dried oregano

1   tsp dried thyme

1   bay leaf

1   can (14 oz/400g) diced
    tomatoes (preferably
    no added salt)

4   cups low-sodium seafood
    or vegetable broth

½   cup dry white wine
    (optional)

½   lb (225g) firm white fish
    (such as cod or haddock),
    cut into bite-sized pieces

½   lb (225g) large shrimp,
    peeled and deveined

½   lb (225g) mussels or clams,
    cleaned and debearded

½   lb (225g) squid rings
    and tentacles

    Salt and pepper, to taste

    Chopped fresh parsley,
    for garnish

    Lemon wedges, for serving

METHOD

1. Heat the olive oil in a large soup pot over medium heat. Add the chopped onion and cook until translucent -about 3-4 minutes.

2. Add the minced garlic, diced red and green bell peppers, and diced carrot, then cook for another 4-5 minutes until the vegetables start to soften.

3. Stir in the smoked paprika, cayenne pepper, dried oregano, dried thyme, and bay leaf. Cook for a minute or two until the spices become fragrant.

4. Add the diced tomatoes, seafood or vegetable broth, and white wine (if using). Bring the mixture to a simmer and let it cook for about 15-20 minutes, allowing the flavors to blend.

5. Once the base of the soup is well-flavored, gently add the bite-sized pieces of white fish, shrimp, mussels or clams, and squid rings and tentacles. Be sure not to overcook the seafood; it should be tender and opaque.

6. Season the soup with salt and pepper to taste. Remember that the seafood broth may contain some natural saltiness.

7. Once the seafood is cooked, discard any mussels or clams that don't open.

8. Serve, garnished with chopped fresh parsley, and accompanied by lemon wedges for squeezing over the soup.

THAI COCONUT SEAFOOD SOUP

SERVINGS: 4 | CALORIES PER SERVING: 235KCAL | TOTAL COOKING TIME: 350 MINS

INGREDIENTS

1   can (14 oz/400g) coconut milk

3   cups seafood broth (you can use vegetable or chicken broth as well)

1   stalk lemongrass, cut into 2-inch pieces and lightly smashed

3-4 kaffir lime leaves, torn into pieces (optional, but highly recommended)

3-4 slices galangal (Thai ginger)

1   small onion, sliced

1-2 Thai red chilies, sliced (adjust to taste)

1   cup mixed seafood (shrimp, squid, mussels, etc.), cleaned and deveined

1   cup sliced mushrooms (straw mushrooms or button mushrooms)

1   medium tomato, cut into wedges

1   tbsp fish sauce (adjust to taste)

1   tbsp lime juice

1   tsp coconut sugar or brown sugar

Fresh cilantro leaves for garnish

Salt to taste

METHOD

1. In a pot, heat the coconut milk over medium heat. Stir gently as the coconut milk heats to prevent it from separating.

2. Add the lemongrass, kaffir lime leaves, and galangal to the pot. Let them simmer gently in the coconut milk for about 5-7 minutes to infuse the flavors.

3. Add the sliced onion and Thai red chilies to the pot. Continue to simmer for another 2-3 minutes until the onions start to soften.

4. Pour in the seafood broth and bring the mixture to a gentle boil. Let it simmer for about 5 minutes to blend the flavors.

5. Add the mixed seafood, sliced mushrooms, and tomato wedges to the pot. Let them cook for about 3-5 minutes until the seafood is cooked through.

6. Season the soup with salt and pepper, fish sauce, lime juice, and coconut sugar. Taste and adjust the seasoning as needed. If you prefer more heat, you can add more Thai red chilies.

7. Once the seafood is cooked and the flavors have blended, remove the pot from the heat. Discard the lemongrass, kaffir lime leaves, and galangal slices.

8. Serve in bowls, garnished with fresh cilantro leaves. You can also add a few extra slices of Thai red chilies for those who enjoy extra spiciness.

9. Enjoy the soup as a comforting and flavorful appetizer or serve it alongside steamed jasmine rice for a complete meal.

Also known as "Tom Kha Talay," this delicious soup combines the richness of coconut milk and aromatic herbs with the freshness of seafood and aromatic Thai spices.

LEMON GARLIC SHRIMP SOUP

SERVINGS: 4 | CALORIES PER SERVING: 205KCAL | TOTAL COOKING TIME: 35 MINS

INGREDIENTS

1   lb (450g) large shrimp, peeled and deveined

2   tbsp olive oil

1   small onion, finely chopped

3   cloves garlic, minced

1   medium carrot, peeled and diced

1   medium zucchini, diced

4   cups low-sodium chicken or vegetable broth

1   tsp dried thyme

1   bay leaf

    Zest and juice of 1 lemon

    Salt and pepper to taste

    Fresh parsley, chopped (for garnish)

METHOD

1. In a large pot, heat the olive oil over medium heat. Add the chopped onion and sauté until translucent.

2. Add the minced garlic and cook for about 1 minute, until fragrant.

3. Add the diced carrot and zucchini to the pot. Sauté for a few minutes until the vegetables start to soften.

4. Pour in the low-sodium chicken or vegetable broth. Add the dried thyme and bay leaf. Bring the mixture to a gentle boil, then reduce the heat to a simmer.

5. Allow the soup to simmer for about 15-20 minutes, or until the vegetables are tender.

6. While the soup is simmering, season the peeled and deveined shrimp with a pinch of salt and pepper.

7. Add the seasoned shrimp to the simmering soup and cook for about 3-5 minutes, or until the shrimp turn pink and opaque.

8. Remove the bay leaf from the soup and discard.

9. Stir in the lemon zest and lemon juice. Taste and adjust the seasoning with more salt and pepper if needed.

10. Ladle into bowls and garnish with chopped fresh parsley.

11. Serve the soup hot with wholegrain bread or a side salad for a complete and healthy meal.

Lemon garlic shrimp soup is packed with protein from the shrimp and the array of nutritious vegetables. The lemon and garlic add a refreshing and zesty twist to the classic soup, making it a perfect option for a wholesome, healthy well-balanced meal.

FISH

SOUP

RECIPES

CREAMY SMOKED TROUT SOUP

SERVINGS: 4 | CALORIES PER SERVING: 180KCAL | TOTAL COOKING TIME: 45 MINS

INGREDIENTS

8 oz (225g) smoked trout fillets, skin and bones removed

1 tbsp olive oil

1 small onion, finely chopped

2 cloves garlic, minced

2 carrots, peeled and chopped

2 potatoes, peeled and diced

4 cups low-sodium fish or vegetable broth

1 bay leaf

1 tsp dried thyme

½ tsp smoked paprika

½ cup plain fat-free Greek yogurt

2 tbsp fresh dill, chopped

2 tbsp fresh chives, chopped

Salt and pepper to taste

Lemon wedges (for garnish, optional)

METHOD

1. In a large pot, heat the olive oil over medium heat. Add the chopped onion, garlic, and carrots. Sauté for about 5 minutes, or until the vegetables start to soften.

2. Add the diced potatoes to the pot and cook for another 2-3 minutes, stirring occasionally.

3. Pour in the low-sodium fish or vegetable broth, and add the bay leaf, dried thyme, and smoked paprika. Stir well.

4. Bring the soup to a boil, then reduce the heat to low, cover, and simmer for about 15-20 minutes, or until the potatoes are tender.

5. While the soup is simmering, use a fork to break the smoked trout into smaller pieces.

6. Once the potatoes are tender, remove the bay leaf from the soup, and then use an immersion blender to purée the soup until smooth. If you don't have an immersion blender, you can carefully transfer the soup in batches to a blender and blend until smooth, then return it to the pot.

7. Stir in the Greek yogurt, fresh dill, and half of the chopped chives. Mix well until the soup is creamy and well combined.

8. Gently fold in the smoked trout pieces, reserving a few for garnish.

9. Season the soup with salt and pepper to taste. Keep in mind that smoked trout can be salty, so you may not need much additional salt.

10. To serve, ladle into bowls and garnish with the remaining chives. If desired, add a squeeze of fresh lemon juice for a burst of freshness.

THAI COCONUT FISH SOUP

SERVINGS: 4 | CALORIES PER SERVING: 225KCAL | TOTAL COOKING TIME: 35 MINS

INGREDIENTS

1   lb (450g) white fish fillets, such as cod or snapper, cut into bite-sized pieces

1   can (14 oz/400g) low fat coconut milk

3   cups chicken or fish broth

2-3 slices galangal or ginger

2   lemongrass stalks, bruised and cut into pieces

3-4 kaffir lime leaves, torn

1   small onion, thinly sliced

2-3 Thai bird's eye chilies, sliced (adjust to taste)

2   tbsp fish sauce

1   tbsp lime juice

1   tsp coconut/fruit/brown sugar or stevia (optional)

1   cup mixed vegetables (such as mushrooms, bell peppers, and baby corn)

Fresh cilantro leaves, for garnish

Salt, to taste

Fresh cilantro and lime wedges, for serving

METHOD

1. In a pot, bring the chicken or fish broth to a gentle simmer. Add the galangal or ginger slices, lemongrass, and kaffir lime leaves. Let it simmer for about 10-15 minutes to infuse the flavors.

2. Add the sliced onions and Thai bird's eye chilies to the broth. Continue to simmer for a few more minutes until the onions are slightly softened.

3. Pour in the coconut milk and stir gently to combine. Let the mixture simmer for another 5-7 minutes.

4. Add the mixed vegetables to the pot and cook until they are tender but still slightly crisp.

5. Season the soup with fish sauce, lime juice, and coconut sugar (if using). Adjust the flavors according to your taste preferences. If you prefer a spicier soup, you can add more Thai bird's eye chilies.

6. Carefully add the fish fillet pieces to the soup and cook until they are opaque and cooked through, about 5-7 minutes.

7. Taste the soup and adjust the seasoning with a pinch of salt if needed.

8. Once the fish is cooked and the flavors are well-balanced, remove the pot from the heat.

9. Serve hot, garnished with fresh cilantro leaves and lime wedges.

10. Enjoy the aromatic and flavorful Thai fish soup on its own or with a side of steamed jasmine rice.

Also known as Tom Kha Pla, you can customize this soup by adding other ingredients like shrimp, tofu, or additional vegetables. This soup is a perfect combination of creamy coconut milk, fragrant herbs, and delicate fish flavors.

LEMON GARLIC TILAPIA SOUP

SERVINGS: 4 | CALORIES PER SERVING: 425KCAL | TOTAL COOKING TIME: 30 MINS

INGREDIENTS

- 4 tilapia fillets, cut into bite-sized pieces
- 2 tbsp olive oil
- 1 small onion, finely chopped
- 4 cloves garlic, minced
- 1 tsp dried thyme
- 1 tsp dried oregano
- 4 cups low-sodium chicken or vegetable broth
- 1 cup diced tomatoes (canned or fresh)
- ½ cup carrots, peeled and sliced into rounds
- ½ cup red bell pepper, chopped
- Juice of 2 lemons
- Zest of 1 lemon
- Salt and black pepper to taste
- Fresh parsley for garnish

METHOD

1. In a large soup pot, heat the olive oil over medium heat. Add the chopped onion and sauté for about 2-3 minutes until they become translucent.

2. Add the minced garlic, dried thyme, and oregano to the onions. Sauté for another minute until the garlic becomes fragrant.

3. Pour in the low-sodium chicken or vegetable broth and bring the mixture to a simmer.

4. Add the diced tomatoes, carrots, and red bell pepper to the pot. Stir well and let it simmer for about 10-15 minutes until the vegetables become tender.

5. Season the soup with salt and black pepper to taste.

6. Carefully add the tilapia pieces to the simmering soup. Let them cook for about 5-7 minutes until the fish turns opaque and flakes easily with a fork.

7. Stir in the lemon juice and lemon zest. Taste the soup and adjust the seasoning, adding more lemon juice if desired.

8. Once the fish is cooked, remove the soup from heat.

9. Ladle into serving bowls and garnish with fresh parsley. Serve hot.

This soup is not only delicious but also packed with lean protein and omega-6 fats and has fewer calories than salmon. The bright citrusy flavor of lemon complements the flavor perfectly. It's a perfect choice for a light and satisfying meal.

SALMON AND SPINACH SOUP

SERVINGS: 4 | CALORIES PER SERVING: 200KCAL | TOTAL COOKING TIME: 35 MINS

INGREDIENTS

2 salmon fillets (about 8 oz/225g each), skin removed

1 tbsp olive oil

1 small onion, finely chopped

2 cloves garlic, minced

1 carrot, peeled and diced

1 celery stalk, diced

4 cups low-sodium chicken or vegetable broth

1 cup water

1 cup diced tomatoes (canned or fresh)

2 cups fresh spinach leaves, chopped

½ cup whole-grain orzo pasta (or any small pasta of your choice)

1 tsp dried thyme

1 tsp dried oregano

Salt and pepper to taste

Lemon slices (for garnish)

Fresh dill or parsley, chopped (for garnish)

METHOD

1. In a large soup pot, heat the olive oil over a medium heat. Add the chopped onion, garlic, carrot, and celery. Sauté for about 5 minutes, or until the vegetables start to soften.

2. Add the dried thyme and oregano to the sautéed vegetables. Stir well to release their flavors.

3. Pour in the chicken or vegetable broth and water. Bring the mixture to a boil.

4. Once the soup is boiling, add the diced tomatoes and orzo pasta. Reduce the heat to a simmer and cook for about 8-10 minutes or until the pasta is almost tender.

5. While the pasta is cooking, cut the salmon fillets into bite-sized pieces.

6. Add the chopped spinach and salmon pieces to the soup. Continue simmering for an additional 5-7 minutes or until the salmon is cooked through and flakes easily with a fork.

7. Taste the soup and season with salt and pepper according to your preference.

8. Ladle into bowls whilst hot. Garnish each serving with a slice or two of lemon and a sprinkle of fresh chopped parsley.

SPICY FISH CURRY SOUP

SERVINGS: 4 | CALORIES PER SERVING: 325KCAL | TOTAL COOKING TIME: 40 MINS

INGREDIENTS

For the Fish Marinade:

1 lb (450g) white fish fillets (such as cod, tilapia, or haddock), cut into bite-sized pieces

1 tbsp lemon juice

½ tsp ground turmeric

½ tsp ground red chili

Salt to taste

For the Soup:

1 tbsp coconut oil

1 onion, finely chopped

2 cloves garlic, minced

1-inch piece of ginger, minced

1 tsp ground cumin

1 tsp ground coriander

½ tsp ground turmeric

½ tsp ground red chili (adjust to taste)

1 can (14 oz/400g) diced tomatoes

1 can (14 oz/400g) coconut milk

3 cups fish or vegetable broth

1 cup mixed vegetables (such as bell peppers, carrots, and peas)

Salt and pepper to taste

Fresh cilantro leaves for garnish

Lemon wedges for serving

METHOD

1. In a bowl, combine the lemon juice, turmeric powder, red chili powder, and salt. Coat the fish pieces with the marinade and let them sit for about 15-20 minutes.

2. In a large pot, heat coconut oil over medium heat. Add the chopped onion and sauté for 2-3 minutes until translucent.

3. Add the minced garlic and ginger to the pot and sauté for about a minute until fragrant. Stir in the ground cumin, coriander, turmeric, and red chili. Cook for another minute.

4. Add the diced tomatoes (with their juice) to the pot and cook for a few minutes until they start to break down. Pour in the coconut milk and stir well to combine.

5. Pour in the fish or vegetable broth and bring the mixture to a simmer. Let it cook for about 10-15 minutes, allowing the flavors to infuse.

6. Gently add the marinated fish pieces and mixed vegetables to the soup. Simmer for an additional 5-7 minutes or until the fish is cooked through and the vegetables are tender.

7. Taste the soup and adjust the seasoning with salt and pepper as needed. Ladle into bowls and garnish with fresh cilantro leaves.

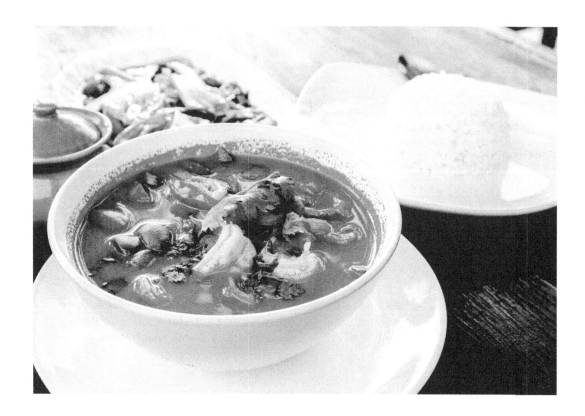

Serve the fish curry soup hot with lemon wedges on the side or a bowl of boiled rice for a more filling meal. The citrusy tang of the lemon juice adds a refreshing contrast to the rich flavors of the soup.

MOROCCAN FISH SOUP

SERVINGS: 4 | CALORIES PER SERVING: 250KCAL | TOTAL COOKING TIME: 40 MINS

INGREDIENTS

1   tbsp olive oil

1   onion, finely chopped

2   garlic cloves, minced

1   tsp ground cumin

1   tsp ground coriander

½   tsp ground paprika

¼   tsp ground turmeric

¼   tsp ground cinnamon

Pinch of cayenne pepper (adjust to taste)

1   can (14 oz) diced tomatoes

4   cups vegetable or fish broth

1   cup water

1   red bell pepper, chopped

1   carrot, peeled and chopped

1   zucchini, chopped

½   cup cooked chickpeas (canned or cooked from dried)

1   lb (450g) white fish fillets (such as cod or haddock), cut into bite-sized chunks

Juice of 1 lemon

Salt and black pepper to taste

Fresh cilantro or parsley, chopped, for garnish

METHOD

1. In a large pot or Dutch oven, heat the olive oil over medium heat and add the chopped onion and sauté until it becomes translucent.

2. Add the minced garlic, ground cumin, ground coriander, ground paprika, ground turmeric, ground cinnamon, and cayenne pepper. Stir well and let the spices cook for a minute until fragrant.

3. Add the can of diced tomatoes (including the liquid) to the pot. Stir to combine with the onion and spices.

4. Pour in the vegetable or fish broth and the water. Stir to combine all the ingredients.

5. Add the chopped red bell pepper, carrot, and zucchini to the pot. Stir well and let the soup come to a gentle simmer.

6. Allow the soup to simmer for about 15-20 minutes, or until the vegetables are tender.

7. Gently add the chunks of white fish and the cooked chickpeas to the soup. Be careful not to over-stir to avoid breaking up the fish.

8. Let the soup simmer for an additional 8-10 minutes, or until the fish is cooked through and flakes easily with a fork.

9. Add the lemon juice to the soup and stir gently. Season the soup with salt and black pepper to taste. Adjust the cayenne pepper if you prefer more heat.

10. Ladle into bowls. Garnish with chopped fresh cilantro or parsley.

11. Serve the soup hot with crusty wholegrain bread or a side of cooked quinoa for a complete and satisfying meal.

VIETNAMESE FISH SOUP

SERVINGS: 4 | CALORIES PER SERVING: 150KCAL | TOTAL COOKING TIME: 40 MINS

INGREDIENTS

For the broth:

4 cups water or fish stock

1 stalk lemongrass, bruised and cut into 2-inch (5cm) pieces

1 small onion, peeled and sliced

1 tomato, cut into wedges

2 cloves garlic, minced

1 thumb-sized piece of ginger, sliced

2-3 kaffir lime leaves (optional)

1 tbsp tamarind paste

1 tbsp fish sauce

For the soup:

½ lb (225g) white fish fillets (such as catfish or tilapia), cut into bite-sized pieces

1 cup mixed vegetables (okra, bean sprouts, zucchini, etc.)

½ cup pineapple chunks

1 red chili pepper, sliced (adjust to your spice preference)

Fresh herbs like cilantro and Thai basil, chopped

Salt and pepper to taste

METHOD

1. In a large pot, bring water or fish stock to a boil.

2. Next, add lemongrass, sliced onion, tomato wedges, minced garlic, ginger slices, and kaffir lime leaves (if using).

3. Let the broth simmer for about 15-20 minutes to infuse the flavors.

4. Stir in the tamarind paste and fish sauce. Adjust the amount of tamarind and fish sauce to your taste preference. Continue to simmer for an additional 5-10 minutes.

5. Strain the broth to remove the solid ingredients, leaving a clear and flavorful broth.

6. Return the strained broth to the pot and bring it back to a gentle simmer.

7. Add the fish fillets, mixed vegetables, and pineapple chunks to the broth.

8. Let the fish cook for about 5-7 minutes or until it's opaque and cooked through.

9. Season the soup with salt and pepper to taste and add the sliced red chili pepper for some heat (adjust to your spice preference).

10. Ladle the soup into serving bowls and sprinkle the chopped fresh herbs (cilantro and Thai basil) over the soup for added freshness and flavor.

Serve the fish soup hot, accompanied by steamed rice or rice noodles if desired.

Often known as "Canh Chua Ca," this soup is also called Vietnamese sweet & sour soup.

It's light, flavorful, and packed with nutritious ingredients. Is has a delightful combination of tangy, savory, and slightly sweet flavors and originates from the Mekong Delta in southern Vietnam where it is classically made with catfish.

ASIAN GINGER FISH SOUP

· ·

SERVINGS: 4 | CALORIES PER SERVING: 200KCAL | TOTAL COOKING TIME: 25 MINS

INGREDIENTS

1 tbsp sesame oil

4 cups fish or vegetable
   broth (low sodium)

1 lb (450g) white fish fillets
   (such as cod or tilapia),
   cut into bite-sized pieces

1 thumb-sized piece of
   fresh ginger, peeled
   and thinly sliced

2 cloves garlic, minced

2 tbsp low-sodium soy sauce

2 heads baby bok
   choy, trimmed and
   leaves separated

4 green onions, thinly sliced

1 red chili pepper, thinly
   sliced (optional, for heat)

1 tbsp rice vinegar

   Salt and pepper to taste

   Fresh cilantro leaves
   for garnish (optional)

METHOD

1. In a large soup pot, heat the sesame oil
    over gentle heat. Add the sliced ginger and
    minced garlic, do not allow to burn. Sauté
    for about 1-2 minutes until fragrant.

2. Pour in the fish or vegetable broth and
    bring it to a gentle simmer. Let it simmer
    for about 10 minutes to infuse the broth
    with ginger and garlic flavors.

3. Add the low-sodium soy sauce and rice
    vinegar to the broth. Stir well to combine.

4. Carefully add the bite-sized pieces of
    white fish to the simmering broth. Cook
    for about 5 minutes, or until the fish is
    opaque and flakes easily with a fork. Be
    careful not to overcook the fish.

5. While the fish is cooking, prepare the bok
    choy. Slice the baby bok choy leaves into
    thin strips and set aside.

6. Once the fish is cooked, taste the soup,
    and season with salt and pepper as
    needed. If you prefer a spicier soup, you
    can add the thinly sliced red chili pepper
    at this stage.

7. Just before serving, add the sliced bok
    choy to the soup. Let it cook for about 2-3
    minutes until the bok choy leaves are
    tender and vibrant green.

8. Stir in most of the sliced green onions,
    reserving a few for garnish.

9. Ladle the soup into bowls, ensuring that
    each serving includes a generous portion
    of fish, bok choy, and broth.

10. Garnish each bowl with the remaining
    sliced green onions and, if desired, fresh
    cilantro leaves.

PORTUGUESE FISH SOUP

SERVINGS: 4 | CALORIES PER SERVING: 250KCAL | TOTAL COOKING TIME: 40 MINS

INGREDIENTS

- 1   tbsp olive oil
- 1   lb (450g) mixed firm fish fillets (such as cod, haddock, or snapper), cut into bite-sized chunks
- ½   lb (225g) small new potatoes, sliced
- 1   onion, finely chopped
- 2   cloves garlic, minced
- 1   red bell pepper, sliced
- 1   green bell pepper, sliced
- 1   tomato, chopped
- ½   cup dry white wine
- 4   cups fish or vegetable broth
- 1   bay leaf
- 1   tsp paprika
- ½   tsp saffron threads (optional)
- ¼   cup chopped fresh parsley
  Salt and pepper to taste

METHOD

1. Heat a large soup pot over medium heat. Add a drizzle of olive oil and sauté the chopped onion and minced garlic until softened and fragrant.

2. Add the sliced bell peppers and chopped tomato to the pot. Cook for a few minutes until the vegetables start to soften.

3. Sprinkle in the paprika and saffron threads (if using). Stir well to combine and release their flavors.

4. Pour in the white wine and let it simmer for a couple of minutes to reduce slightly.

5. Add the sliced potatoes and bay leaf to the pot. Pour in the fish or vegetable broth, making sure the potatoes are submerged. If needed, add a bit more water to cover the ingredients.

6. Season with salt and pepper to taste. Remember that the broth will reduce, so you can adjust the seasoning later if necessary.

7. Bring the soup to a gentle simmer and cook for about 15-20 minutes, or until the potatoes are tender.

8. Carefully add the chunks of fish to the soup. Make sure they are submerged in the broth. Cook for an additional 5-7 minutes, or until the fish is cooked through and flakes easily.

9. Taste the soup and adjust the seasoning if needed. Remove the bay leaf.

10. Ladle the soup into bowls, ensuring each serving has a good mixture of fish, vegetables, and potatoes.

11. Garnish the soup with chopped fresh parsley for a burst of color and flavor.

12. Serve, accompanied by crusty bread or a side of cooked rice if desired.

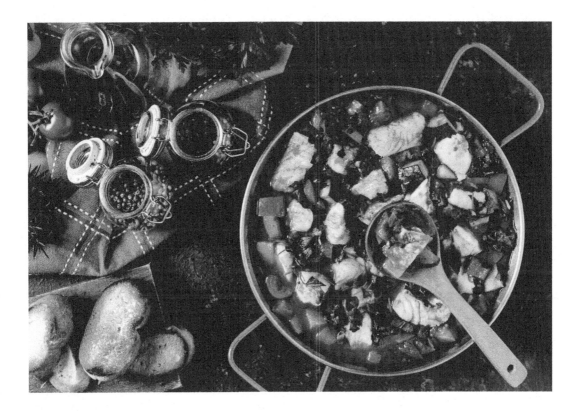

Also known as "Caldeirada de Peixe," this flavorful soup is a traditional Portuguese dish that combines fresh fish with vegetables, spices, and aromatic herbs in a rich broth. It's a nourishing and delicious option for seafood lovers that was created by fishermen needing a fulfilling meal after a hard day's work.

ITALIAN FISH SOUP

SERVINGS: 4 | CALORIES PER SERVING: 175KCAL | TOTAL COOKING TIME: 30 MINS

INGREDIENTS

- 2 tbsp olive oil
- 1 lb (450g) mixed firm white fish fillets (such as cod, haddock, or snapper), cut into chunks
- ½ lb (225g) medium shrimp, peeled and deveined
- ½ lb (225g) mussels, cleaned and debearded
- ½ lb (225g) clams, scrubbed and cleaned
- ¼ cup olive oil
- 1 onion, finely chopped
- 3 garlic cloves, minced
- 1 red bell pepper, diced
- 1 yellow bell pepper, diced
- 1 celery stalk, diced
- 1 carrot, peeled and diced
- 1 can (14 oz/400g) diced tomatoes, with juices
- 4 cups fish or seafood broth
- ½ cup dry white wine (optional)
- ½ tsp red pepper flakes (adjust to taste)
- 1 tsp dried oregano
- 1 tsp dried thyme
- Salt and pepper to taste
- Fresh basil and parsley, chopped, for garnish
- Lemon wedges, for serving

METHOD

1. In a large soup pot or Dutch oven, heat the olive oil over medium heat.

2. Add the chopped onion, garlic, diced red and yellow bell peppers, celery, and carrot. Sauté for about 5-7 minutes until the vegetables soften and become aromatic.

3. Stir in the canned diced tomatoes, dried oregano, dried thyme, red pepper flakes, salt, and pepper. Cook for a few minutes to allow the flavors to infuse.

4. If using white wine, pour it into the pot and let it simmer for a couple of minutes to cook off the alcohol.

5. Pour in the fish or seafood broth. Bring the mixture to a simmer and let it cook for about 15-20 minutes, allowing the flavors to develop.

6. Gently add the fish chunks, shrimp, mussels, and clams to the pot. Make sure the seafood is submerged in the broth. Cover the pot and let the seafood cook for about 5-7 minutes until the fish is opaque, shrimp are pink, and the mussels and clams have opened. Discard any mussels or clams that remain closed.

7. Taste the soup and adjust the seasoning with more salt and pepper if needed.

8. Ladle the soup into bowls, making sure each serving has a good variety of the seafood. Garnish with chopped fresh basil and parsley. Serve with lemon wedges on the side.

This Italian Fish Soup is commonly known as "Zuppa di Pesce." It's packed with flavor and is very nutritious as it is rich in protein, vitamins, and minerals from the seafood and vegetables. It is one of the classic seafood soup recipes and distinctive as it is tomato-based. It's a perfect dish for enjoying the flavors of the Mediterranean in a wholesome and satisfying way.

. . . .

Bulk Up with Beans: Beans add protein and fiber. Use varieties like black beans, lentils, or chickpeas.

. . . .

. . . .

Watch Portions: Use smaller portions of high-calorie ingredients like cheese or cream.

. . . .

. . . .

Use low-fat yogurt or milk instead of heavy cream for creamy soups.

. . . .

FISHERMAN'S SOUP

SERVINGS: 4 | CALORIES PER SERVING: 190KCAL | TOTAL COOKING TIME: 55 MINS

INGREDIENTS

1   tbsp olive oil

1   large onion, peeled, finely chopped

1   bulb fennel, finely chopped

1   carrot, peeled and finely chopped

5   garlic cloves, crushed and finely chopped

2   sprigs fresh thyme

1   fresh bay leaf

Pinch saffron, ground to a powder in a mortar and pestle

½   lb (250g) red snapper, skin and bones removed, flesh chopped into small pieces

½   lb (250g) grey mullet, skin and bones removed, chopped into small pieces

1   can (14 oz/400g) chopped tomatoes

2   cups dry white wine (optional)

2   cups low sodium fish or vegetable broth

1   pinch cayenne pepper

Salt and pepper to taste

Fresh cilantro or parsley, chopped, for garnish

Juice of ½ lemon

METHOD

1. Heat the oil in a large soup pot over a medium heat, add the onions, fennel, carrot, garlic, thyme sprigs and bay leaf and fry gently for 4-5 minutes, stirring well, until the vegetables have softened.

2. Add the saffron and stir well, then add the fish pieces and stir again. Continue to cook for a further 4-5 minutes.

3. If using white wine, pour it into the pot and let it simmer for a couple of minutes to cook off the alcohol.

4. Add the tomatoes and broth, then season, to taste, with the sea salt and cayenne pepper.

5. Bring the mixture to the boil and boil for 2-3 minutes. Skim off any foam from the surface of the water, then reduce the heat to low and simmer gently for 20-25 minutes. Remove from the heat and set aside to cool slightly.

6. Blend in a food processor to a rough purée, according to your taste preference.

7. Season the soup with salt and black pepper to taste. Remember that the seafood broth may already be salty, so adjust accordingly. Remove the bay leaf from the soup.

8. Ladle into bowls and garnish with chopped fresh parsley or cilantro and a squeeze of lemon juice.

MEXICAN FISH SOUP

· ·

SERVINGS: 4 | CALORIES PER SERVING: 200KCAL | TOTAL COOKING TIME: 40 MINS

INGREDIENTS

- 1 tbsp olive oil
- 1 lb (450g) white fish fillets (such as cod, tilapia, or snapper), cut into bite-sized pieces
- 1 onion, chopped
- 2 cloves garlic, minced
- 1 bell pepper, diced
- 2 medium tomatoes, chopped
- 1 zucchini, sliced
- 1 carrot, peeled and sliced
- 4 cups fish or vegetable broth
- 1 cup water
- 1 tsp ground cumin
- 1 tsp chili powder (adjust to taste)
- ½ tsp paprika
- ¼ tsp cayenne pepper (adjust to taste)
- Salt and black pepper to taste
- Juice of 1 lime
- Fresh cilantro, chopped, for garnish
- Sliced avocado, for garnish
- Lime wedges, for serving

METHOD

1. Heat a large pot over a medium heat. Add the olive oil and sauté the chopped onion and minced garlic until fragrant and translucent.

2. Add the diced bell pepper, chopped tomatoes, sliced zucchini, and sliced carrot to the pot. Sauté for a few minutes until the vegetables begin to soften.

3. Pour in the fish or vegetable broth and water. Stir in the ground cumin, chili powder, paprika, and cayenne pepper. Season with salt and black pepper to taste.

4. Bring the soup to a gentle simmer and let it cook for about 15-20 minutes, or until the vegetables are tender.

5. Gently add the bite-sized fish fillet pieces to the simmering soup. Be careful not to over-stir to prevent the fish from breaking apart. Cook for another 5-7 minutes, or until the fish is opaque and fully cooked.

6. Squeeze the juice of one lime into the soup and stir to incorporate.

7. Taste the soup and adjust the seasonings, if needed, by adding more chili powder, cayenne pepper, salt, or lime juice.

8. Ladle the hot soup into serving bowls and garnish with chopped fresh cilantro, sliced avocado, and lime wedges on the side.

Known in Mexico as "Caldo de Pescado," this flavorful and nutritious soup is packed with fresh vegetables and delicious fish, making it a perfect choice for a light and satisfying meal.

JAPANESE MISO FISH SOUP

SERVINGS: 2 | CALORIES PER SERVING: 220KCAL | TOTAL COOKING TIME: 30 MINS

INGREDIENTS

2   cups water

2   cups fish or vegetable broth

2   tbsp miso paste
    (white or red)

1   small onion, thinly sliced

2   cloves garlic, minced

1   small carrot, peeled
    and julienned

1   cup sliced mushrooms
    (shiitake or oyster
    mushrooms work well)

1   cup baby spinach or
    chopped spinach leaves

8   oz (225g) firm white
    fish fillets (such as cod
    or haddock), cut into
    bite-sized pieces

2   green onions, sliced
    (for garnish)

1   tbsp soy sauce
    (low sodium)

1   tbsp rice vinegar

1   tsp sesame oil

    Optional toppings:
    toasted sesame seeds,
    sliced nori seaweed

METHOD

1. In a pot, bring the water and fish or vegetable broth to a gentle simmer over medium heat.

2. Add the sliced onion and minced garlic to the simmering broth. Let them cook for a few minutes until they start to soften.

3. Stir in the julienned carrot and sliced mushrooms. Let the vegetables cook for another 3-4 minutes until they begin to soften.

4. In a small bowl, dilute the miso paste with a little of the hot broth to create a smooth mixture. This step prevents the miso from forming lumps when added to the soup. Gradually add the diluted miso paste to the pot, stirring gently to incorporate it into the soup.

5. Carefully add the fish fillet pieces into the simmering broth. Let them cook for about 5-7 minutes, or until cooked through and flakes easily with a fork.

6. Stir in the soy sauce, rice vinegar, and sesame oil. Taste the soup and adjust the seasoning if needed.

7. Just before serving, add the baby spinach to the pot. It will wilt quickly in the hot broth.

8. Ladle the hot miso fish soup into bowls. Garnish with sliced green onions and, if desired, sprinkle with toasted sesame seeds and sliced nori seaweed.

Miso paste is salty, so there's usually no need to add extra salt to the soup. The amount of miso paste used can be adjusted according to your taste preferences. You can also customize this recipe by adding other vegetables like bok choy, snow peas, or corn.

Remember that miso paste also contains beneficial probiotics, which are good for gut health.

CARIBBEAN FISH SOUP

SERVINGS: 4 | CALORIES PER SERVING: 225KCAL | TOTAL COOKING TIME: 40 MINS

INGREDIENTS

1   lb (450g) white fish fillets (such as snapper, cod, or grouper), cut into bite-sized chunks

1   tbsp olive oil

1   onion, chopped

2   cloves garlic, minced

1   bell pepper, sliced

1   carrot, peeled and sliced

1   celery stalk, sliced

1   medium potato, diced

1   cup diced tomatoes (fresh or canned)

4   cups fish or vegetable broth

1   cup coconut milk (light or full fat)

1   tsp ground cumin

1   tsp ground coriander

1   tsp paprika

½   tsp turmeric

¼   tsp cayenne pepper (adjust to taste)

Salt and black pepper to taste

Juice of 1 lime

Fresh cilantro or parsley, chopped (for garnish)

Sliced scallions (for garnish)

METHOD

1. Heat the olive oil in a large soup pot over medium heat. Add the chopped onion and sauté for a few minutes until it becomes translucent.

2. Add the minced garlic, diced bell pepper, carrot, celery, and diced potato to the pot. Sauté for another few minutes until the vegetables start to soften.

3. Stir in the ground cumin, ground coriander, paprika, turmeric, and cayenne pepper. Let the spices cook for a minute to release their flavors.

4. Add the diced tomatoes to the pot and stir to combine. Cook for a couple more minutes to allow the tomatoes to break down slightly.

5. Pour in the fish or vegetable broth and bring the mixture to a gentle simmer. Let it cook for about 10-15 minutes, or until the vegetables are tender. You can blend the soup at this stage if you wish but reserve a few slices of the cooked red pepper for garnish.

6. Gently add the chunks of fish to the simmering soup. Cook for about 5-7 minutes, or until the fish is cooked through and flakes easily with a fork.

7. Stir in the coconut milk and lime juice. Allow the flavors to blend for a few more minutes. Season the soup with salt and black pepper to taste.

8. Taste the soup and adjust the seasoning or spiciness if needed.

9. Ladle the soup into serving bowls. Garnish each bowl with chopped cilantro or parsley and sliced scallions and the reserved red pepper slices.

10. Serve the soup hot with some crusty wholegrain bread or steamed rice on the side.

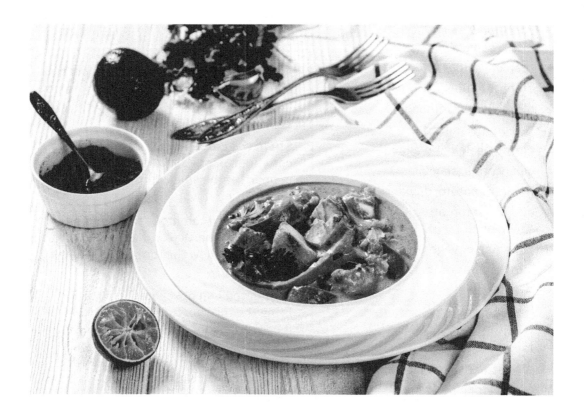

In the Caribbean, fish soup is also known as 'Fish Tea'. Rich in protein, vegetables, and exotic spices, this is a delightful and healthy dish that captures the essence of the Caribbean cuisine.

SCANDINAVIAN FISH SOUP

SERVINGS: 4 | CALORIES PER SERVING: 300KCAL | TOTAL COOKING TIME: 40 MINS

INGREDIENTS

- 1 lb (450g) white fish fillets (such as cod or haddock), cut into bite-sized pieces
- 1 onion, finely chopped
- 2 carrots, peeled and sliced
- 2 celery stalks, sliced
- 2 potatoes, peeled and diced
- 2 cloves garlic, minced
- 1 leek, cleaned and sliced
- 4 cups fish or vegetable broth
- 1 cup low-fat milk or unsweetened almond or low-fat coconut milk
- ½ cup dry white wine (optional)
- 1 bay leaf
- 1 tsp dried dill
- ½ tsp dried thyme
- Salt and pepper, to taste
- 2 tbsp olive oil
- Fresh dill, for garnish
- Lemon wedges, for serving

METHOD

1. Heat the olive oil in a large pot over medium heat. Add the chopped onion, carrots, celery, leek, and garlic. Sauté for a few minutes until the vegetables start to soften.

2. Pour in the white wine (if using) and let it simmer for a couple of minutes to reduce slightly.

3. Add the diced potatoes, bay leaf, dried dill, and dried thyme to the pot. Season with a pinch of salt and pepper. Stir well to combine.

4. Pour in the fish or vegetable broth. Bring the mixture to a gentle simmer and let it cook for about 15-20 minutes, or until the potatoes are tender.

5. Once the potatoes are cooked, reduce the heat to low and add the fish pieces to the pot. Simmer gently for about 5-7 minutes, or until the fish is cooked through and flakes easily with a fork.

6. Pour in the low-fat milk or almond milk and stir gently to combine. Let the soup warm through, but do not let it boil.

7. Taste and adjust the seasoning with additional salt and pepper, if needed.

8. Remove the bay leaf from the soup.

9. To serve, ladle into bowls. Garnish with fresh dill and a squeeze of lemon juice.

10. Serve the soup with wholegrain bread or crispbread on the side for a complete meal.

VEGETABLE SOUP RECIPE

CLASSIC VEGETABLE SOUP

· ·

SERVINGS: 4 | CALORIES PER SERVING: 150KCAL | TOTAL COOKING TIME: 40 MINS

INGREDIENTS

- 1 tbsp olive oil
- 1 onion, chopped
- 2 cloves garlic, minced
- 3 carrots, peeled and chopped
- 1 red bell pepper, chopped
- 1 zucchini, chopped
- 1 cup green beans, chopped
- 1 can (14 oz/400g) diced tomatoes
- 6 cups vegetable broth (low sodium)
- 1 tsp dried thyme
- 1 tsp dried oregano
- 1 bay leaf
- Salt and pepper to taste
- 2 cups baby spinach or kale, chopped
- Fresh parsley, chopped (for garnish)

METHOD

1. Heat the olive oil in a large pot over medium heat. Add the chopped onion and sauté for about 2-3 minutes, until translucent.

2. Add the minced garlic and sauté for an additional 30 seconds, until fragrant.

3. Add the chopped carrots, red bell pepper, zucchini, and green beans to the pot. Sauté for about 5 minutes, stirring occasionally, until the vegetables start to soften.

4. Pour in the diced tomatoes (with their juice) and vegetable broth. Add the dried thyme, dried oregano, bay leaf, and season with salt and pepper to taste.

5. Bring the soup to a boil, then reduce the heat to low. Cover the pot and let the soup simmer for about 20-25 minutes, until the vegetables are tender.

6. Once the vegetables are cooked, remove the bay leaf from the pot.

7. Stir in the chopped baby spinach or kale and let it wilt into the soup for a few minutes.

8. Taste and adjust the seasoning if needed.

9. Ladle the soup into bowls and garnish with freshly chopped parsley.

10. Serve warm and enjoy as a nutritious and comforting meal.

You can switch up this recipe by adding other vegetables of your choice, such as corn, peas, or potatoes. You can also add a squeeze of lemon juice for a burst of freshness. This soup is not only delicious but also packed with vitamins, minerals, and fiber from the variety of vegetables.

MINESTRONE SOUP

SERVINGS: 6 | CALORIES PER SERVING: 175KCAL | TOTAL COOKING TIME: 40 MINS

INGREDIENTS

2   tbsp olive oil

1   onion, chopped

2   carrots, peeled and diced

2   celery stalks, diced

3   cloves garlic, minced

1   zucchini, diced

1   yellow bell pepper, diced

1   tsp dried oregano

1   tsp dried basil

½   tsp dried thyme

½   tsp dried rosemary

½   tsp red pepper flakes
    (adjust to taste)

1   can (14 oz/400g)
    diced tomatoes

6   cups vegetable broth

1   can (14 oz/400g) cannellini
    beans, drained and rinsed

½   cup whole wheat or
    gluten-free pasta

1   cup chopped fresh
    spinach or kale

    Salt and pepper to taste

    Grated Parmesan cheese
    (optional, for serving)

    Fresh chopped parsley
    (for garnish)

METHOD

1. Heat olive oil in a large pot over medium heat. Add chopped onion, diced carrots, and diced celery. Sauté for about 5 minutes until the vegetables start to soften.

2. Add minced garlic, diced zucchini, and diced yellow bell pepper to the pot. Sauté for an additional 3-4 minutes.

3. Stir in the dried oregano, basil, thyme, rosemary, and red pepper flakes. Cook for a minute or two until the herbs are fragrant.

4. Add the diced tomatoes (with their juice) to the pot. Stir well to combine the flavors.

5. Pour in the vegetable broth and bring the mixture to a boil. Once boiling, reduce the heat to low and let the soup simmer for about 15-20 minutes.

6. Add the drained and rinsed cannellini beans to the pot. Stir in the pasta and let the soup simmer for another 10-12 minutes, or until the pasta is cooked.

7. Toss in the chopped spinach or kale and let it wilt into the soup.

8. Taste the soup and season with salt and pepper according to your preference.

9. Once the pasta is tender and the vegetables are cooked to your liking, remove the pot from the heat.

10. Ladle the soup into bowls. If desired, top each bowl with a sprinkle of grated Parmesan cheese and fresh chopped parsley.

11. Serve with whole grain bread or a side salad for a complete and hearty meal.

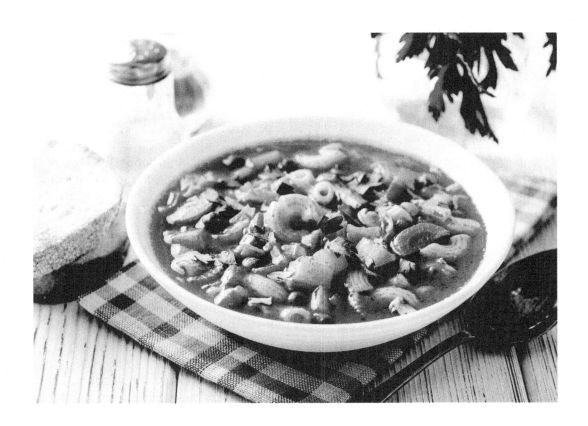

Roasting vegetables before adding to the soup intensifies their taste without added calories.

A squeeze of lemon or lime adds brightness without extra salt.

Use low-sodium soy sauce and broths to control sodium intake.

LENTIL AND VEGETABLE SOUP

SERVINGS: 6 | CALORIES PER SERVING: 120KCAL | TOTAL COOKING TIME: 40 MINS

INGREDIENTS

- 1 cup dried green or brown lentils, rinsed and drained
- 1 tbsp olive oil
- 1 onion, chopped
- 2 carrots, peeled and diced
- 2 cloves garlic, minced
- 1 tsp ground cumin
- ½ tsp ground coriander
- ½ tsp smoked paprika
- ¼ tsp red pepper flakes (adjust to taste)
- 6 cups low-sodium vegetable broth
- 1 can (14 oz/400g) diced tomatoes
- 2 bay leaves
- 2 cups chopped kale or spinach
- Salt and pepper, to taste
- Fresh lemon juice, for serving
- Chopped fresh parsley or cilantro, for garnish

Lentil and vegetable soup is not only nutritious, but also versatile and comforting, making it a perfect option for a healthy meal.

METHOD

1. Heat the olive oil in a large pot or Dutch oven over medium heat. Add the chopped onion, and carrots. Cook for about 5-7 minutes, or until the vegetables start to soften.

2. Add the minced garlic, ground cumin, ground coriander, smoked paprika, and red pepper flakes. Cook for an additional 1-2 minutes, stirring constantly, until the spices are fragrant.

3. Add the rinsed lentils to the pot and stir to coat them with the spices and vegetables.

4. Pour in the vegetable broth and diced tomatoes (with their juices). Add the bay leaves. Bring the mixture to a boil, then reduce the heat to low, cover the pot, and let it simmer for about 20-25 minutes, or until the lentils are tender.

5. Once the lentils are cooked, add the chopped kale or spinach to the pot. Stir and let the greens wilt in the soup.

6. Remove the bay leaves and discard them. Taste the soup and season with salt and pepper to your preference.

7. If desired, use an immersion blender to partially blend the soup. This will help thicken the soup slightly while still leaving some texture from the vegetables and lentils. Alternatively, you can transfer a portion of the soup to a blender, blend until smooth, and then return it to the pot.

8. Just before serving, squeeze fresh lemon juice into the soup for a burst of brightness and flavor.

9. Ladle into bowls and garnish with chopped fresh parsley or cilantro.

10. Serve hot with wholegrain bread or a side salad for a complete and satisfying meal.

BUTTERNUT SQUASH SOUP

SERVINGS: 4 | CALORIES PER SERVING: 125KCAL | TOTAL COOKING TIME: 35 MINS

INGREDIENTS

1   medium butternut squash, peeled, seeded, and cubed

1   onion, chopped

2   carrots, peeled and chopped

2   cloves garlic, minced

1   apple, peeled, cored, and chopped

4   cups vegetable broth

½   tsp ground ginger

½   tsp ground cinnamon

¼   tsp ground nutmeg

Salt and pepper to taste

2   tbsp olive oil

Optional toppings: Fat-free Greek yogurt, pumpkin seeds, chopped fresh herbs

This soup is not only comforting and flavorful but also packed with nutrients from the butternut squash and other wholesome ingredients. It's a perfect dish for cooler days or whenever you're craving a nourishing, warming bowl of soup.

METHOD

1. Heat the olive oil in a large pot over medium heat. Add the chopped onion, carrots, and garlic. Sauté for about 5 minutes, or until the vegetables are slightly softened.

2. Add the chopped butternut squash and apple to the pot. Cook for another 5 minutes, stirring occasionally.

3. Pour in the vegetable broth and bring the mixture to a boil. Reduce the heat to low, cover the pot, and let it simmer for about 20-25 minutes, or until the squash is tender.

4. Using an immersion blender or a regular blender, carefully blend the soup until smooth and creamy. If using a regular blender, blend in batches and return the soup to the pot.

5. Add the ground ginger, cinnamon, nutmeg, salt, and pepper to the soup. Stir well to combine the flavors.

6. Taste the soup and adjust the seasonings as needed. If the soup is too thick, you can add a little more vegetable broth or water to achieve your desired consistency.

7. Once the soup is heated through and seasoned to your liking, remove it from the heat.

8. Serve hot. You can garnish each serving with a dollop of fat-free Greek yogurt, a sprinkle of pumpkin seeds, and some chopped fresh herbs like parsley or chives.

9. Serve and enjoy!

ROASTED TOMATO AND BASIL SOUP

SERVINGS: 4 | CALORIES PER SERVING: 135KCAL | TOTAL COOKING TIME: 60 MINS

INGREDIENTS

1-2 tbsp olive oil

8-10 ripe tomatoes, halved

1   onion, roughly chopped

4   cloves garlic, minced

2   tablespoons olive oil

Salt and black pepper to taste

1   tsp coconut or fruit sugar (optional, to balance acidity)

¼ cup fresh basil leaves, plus extra for garnish

4   cups vegetable broth (or chicken broth for a non-vegetarian version)

½ cup low fat coconut milk (optional, for a creamier soup)

Croutons for garnish (optional)

METHOD

1.   Preheat your oven to 400°F (200°C).

2.   Place the halved tomatoes on a baking sheet, cut side up and drizzle a little olive oil over them.

3.   Sprinkle minced garlic and chopped onion evenly over the tomatoes, then season with salt and black pepper. If your tomatoes are very acidic, sprinkle a teaspoon of coconut or fruit sugar over them to balance the flavors.

4.   Roast the tomatoes in the preheated oven for about 30-40 minutes, or until they become tender and start to caramelize at the edges. The roasting time may vary depending on the size and ripeness of your tomatoes.

5.   Remove the roasted tomatoes, garlic, and onions from the oven and transfer them to a blender or food processor.

6.   Add the fresh basil leaves to the blender and pulse until you have a smooth purée. You may need to do this in batches.

7.   Pour the tomato mixture into a large pot and add the vegetable or chicken broth and stir well.

8.   Heat the soup over medium heat, stirring occasionally, until it's heated through.

9.   If you want a creamier soup, stir in the low-fat coconut milk at this stage. You can adjust the amount to your liking. If the soup is too thick, you can add a bit more broth to reach your desired consistency.

10.   Taste the soup and adjust the seasoning with additional salt and pepper if needed. Let the soup simmer for another 5-10 minutes to allow the flavors to blend together.

11.   Garnish each bowl with fresh basil leaves, and croutons if desired and serve.

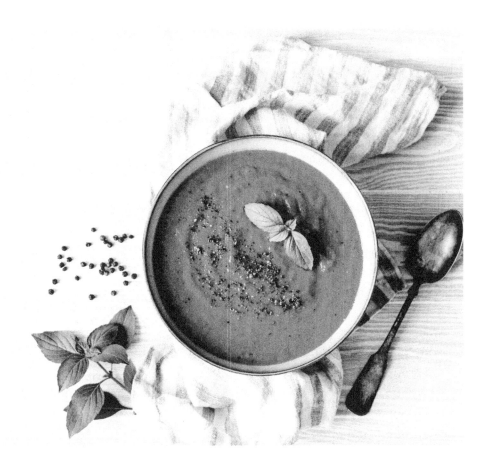

This soup is a delightful way to savor the rich, natural flavors of ripe tomatoes and fresh basil. It's perfect as an appetizer or a light meal and pairs wonderfully with a slice of crusty bread or toasted potato cake.

SWEET POTATO AND KALE SOUP

SERVINGS: 4 | CALORIES PER SERVING: 150KCAL | TOTAL COOKING TIME: 40 MINS

INGREDIENTS

2 medium sweet potatoes, peeled and diced

1 bunch kale, stems removed and chopped

1 onion, chopped

2 cloves garlic, minced

1 carrot, peeled and diced

1 celery stalk, diced

4 cups vegetable broth

1 cup coconut milk (or other plant-based milk)

1 tsp ground cumin

½ tsp ground turmeric

½ tsp ground ginger

¼ tsp ground cinnamon

Salt and pepper to taste

2 tbsp olive oil

Optional toppings:
chopped fresh herbs, pumpkin seeds, and a drizzle of olive oil

METHOD

1. Heat the olive oil in a large pot over medium heat. Add the chopped onion and sauté until translucent, which should take around 3-4 minutes.

2. Add the minced garlic, ground cumin, ground turmeric, ground ginger, and ground cinnamon to the pot. Sauté for another 1-2 minutes until fragrant.

3. Add the diced sweet potatoes, carrot, and celery to the pot. Stir to coat the vegetables with the spices and sauté for a few minutes.

4. Pour in the vegetable broth and bring the mixture to a boil. Reduce the heat to low, cover the pot, and let it simmer for about 15-20 minutes, or until the sweet potatoes are tender.

5. Using an immersion blender or a regular blender, carefully blend the soup until smooth and creamy. If using a regular blender, work in batches and allow the soup to cool slightly before blending.

6. Return the blended soup to the pot over low heat. Stir in the coconut milk and chopped kale. Let the soup simmer for an additional 5-7 minutes, or until the kale is wilted and tender.

7. Season the soup with salt and pepper to taste. Adjust the seasoning and spices according to your preference.

8. Once the soup is heated through and the kale is cooked, remove the pot from the heat.

9. Ladle the soup into bowls. Garnish with your choice of toppings, such as chopped fresh herbs, pumpkin seeds, or a drizzle of olive oil.

MUSHROOM BARLEY SOUP

· ·

SERVINGS: 6 | CALORIES PER SERVING: 130KCAL | TOTAL COOKING TIME: 60 MINS

INGREDIENTS

1 cup pearl barley,
   rinsed and drained

8 cups vegetable or mushroom
   broth (low sodium)

2 tbsp olive oil

1 onion, finely chopped

3 cloves garlic, minced

3 carrots, peeled and diced

2 celery stalks, diced

10 oz (about 2 cups)
   mushrooms, sliced

1 tsp dried thyme

1 tsp dried rosemary

1 bay leaf

   Salt and pepper to taste

   Fresh parsley, chopped
   (for garnish)

METHOD

1. Heat the olive oil in a large pot over medium heat. Add the chopped onion and sauté until translucent for around 3-4 minutes.

2. Add the minced garlic, diced carrots, and diced celery to the pot. Sauté for an additional 2-3 minutes until the vegetables start to soften.

3. Add the sliced mushrooms to the pot and cook for about 5-6 minutes, until they release their moisture and start to brown.

4. Stir in the rinsed pearl barley, dried thyme, dried rosemary, and bay leaf. Cook for another 2-3 minutes, allowing the flavors to blend together.

5. Pour in the vegetable or mushroom broth. Bring the soup to a boil, then reduce the heat to low, cover, and let it simmer for about 40-45 minutes, or until the barley is tender.

6. Season the soup with salt and pepper to taste. Remember that the broth might already have some salt, so adjust accordingly.

7. Once the barley is cooked and the flavors have developed, remove the bay leaf.

8. Ladle the mushroom barley soup into bowls. Garnish with chopped fresh parsley for added freshness and color.

9. Serve the soup warm with a slice of wholegrain bread or a side salad if desired.

This recipe provides a delightful blend of earthy mushrooms, hearty barley, and aromatic herbs in a comforting broth. It's a perfect option for a hearty and nutritious meal.

THAI COCONUT VEGETABLE SOUP

SERVINGS: 4 | CALORIES PER SERVING: 250KCAL | TOTAL COOKING TIME: 35 MINS

INGREDIENTS

1 tbsp coconut oil

1 onion, chopped

2 cloves garlic, minced

1 tbsp fresh ginger, grated

2 tbsp Thai red curry paste (adjust to taste)

4 cups vegetable broth

1 can (14 oz/400g) coconut milk (full-fat or light)

2 carrots, peeled and sliced

1 red bell pepper, sliced

1 zucchini, sliced

1 cup broccoli florets

1 cup cauliflower florets

1 cup baby spinach

Juice of 1 lime

2 tbsp soy sauce or tamari (for a gluten-free option)

1 tbsp brown sugar or coconut sugar

Salt and pepper to taste

Fresh cilantro leaves, chopped (for garnish)

Lime wedges (for serving)

METHOD

1. Heat the coconut oil in a large pot over medium heat. Add the chopped onion and cook until translucent.

2. Add the minced garlic and grated ginger to the pot and sauté for about 1 minute, until fragrant.

3. Stir in the Thai red curry paste and cook for another minute, mixing well with the other ingredients.

4. Pour in the vegetable broth and coconut milk. Stir to combine and heat the mixture to a gentle simmer.

5. Add the sliced carrots, red bell pepper, zucchini, broccoli, and cauliflower to the pot. Let the soup simmer for about 10-15 minutes, or until the vegetables are tender.

6. Add the baby spinach to the soup and let it wilt in the hot liquid.

7. In a small bowl, mix together the lime juice, soy sauce or tamari, and sugar. Add this mixture to the soup and stir well. Adjust the seasoning with salt and pepper to taste.

8. Once all the flavors are well combined and the vegetables are cooked to your liking, remove the pot from the heat.

9. Serve the soup hot, garnished with chopped cilantro leaves and lime wedges on the side.

You can adjust this recipe by adding your favorite vegetables, increasing the level of spiciness with the curry paste, or adding protein sources like tofu or cooked chicken. This soup is a comforting and flavorful dish that's perfect for a cozy meal.

GAZPACHO

SERVINGS: 4 | CALORIES PER SERVING: 200KCAL | TOTAL COOKING TIME: 20 MINS

INGREDIENTS

6   ripe tomatoes, cored and chopped

1   cucumber, peeled, seeded, and chopped

1   red bell pepper, seeded and chopped

1   small red onion, chopped

2   cloves garlic, minced

3   cups tomato juice or vegetable broth

¼   cup extra-virgin olive oil

2   tbsp red wine vinegar

1   tsp salt, or to taste

½   tsp black pepper, or to taste

1   tsp dried oregano or basil

Fresh herbs (such as parsley or basil), for garnish

Optional toppings:
diced cucumber, bell pepper, red onion

Gazpacho is a classic cold soup made with uncooked blended vegetables and popular in both Spain and Portugal. Gazpacho is incredibly versatile and can be customized to your taste preferences by adding other fresh vegetables or herbs that you enjoy.

METHOD

1. In a food processor or blender, combine the chopped tomatoes, cucumber, red bell pepper, red onion, and minced garlic. Pulse until the vegetables are finely chopped but not pureed. You can also do this in batches if your blender is small.

2. Add half of the tomato juice or vegetable broth to the blended vegetables. Blend until the mixture becomes smooth and well combined.

3. Depending on your preference, you can leave the gazpacho slightly chunky or blend until completely smooth. If the mixture is too thick, you can add more tomato juice or vegetable broth to achieve the desired consistency.

4. Stir in the extra-virgin olive oil, red wine vinegar, salt, black pepper, and dried oregano or basil. Taste and adjust the seasoning as needed. Gazpacho is traditionally served chilled, so keep in mind that the flavors will blend together and develop as it cools.

5. Transfer the gazpacho to a large bowl or pitcher and cover it. Place it in the refrigerator to chill for at least 2 hours.

6. Before serving, give the gazpacho a good stir. Ladle the chilled soup into bowls and garnish with fresh herbs, such as chopped parsley or basil. You can also add diced cucumber, bell pepper, and red onion as additional toppings.

7. Serve as a light and refreshing appetizer or a main course on hot summer days. It's perfect for a healthy and hydrating meal.

MEXICAN VEGETABLE SOUP

SERVINGS: 6 | CALORIES PER SERVING: 175KCAL | TOTAL COOKING TIME: 35 MINS

INGREDIENTS

- 1 tbsp olive oil
- 1 onion, diced
- 2 cloves garlic, minced
- 1 bell pepper, diced (any color)
- 1 zucchini, diced
- 1 carrot, peeled and diced
- 1 cup corn kernels (fresh, frozen, or canned)
- 1 can (14 oz/400g) black beans, drained and rinsed
- 1 can (14 oz/400g) diced tomatoes
- 4 cups vegetable broth
- 1 tsp ground cumin
- 1 tsp chili powder (adjust to taste)
- ½ tsp paprika
- ½ tsp dried oregano
- Salt and pepper to taste
- Juice of 1 lime
- Fresh cilantro, chopped, for garnish
- Avocado slices, for serving (optional)

METHOD

1. Heat the olive oil in a large pot over medium heat. Add the diced onion and sauté until translucent, about 3-4 minutes.

2. Add the minced garlic, diced bell pepper, zucchini, and carrot. Sauté for another 5 minutes, or until the vegetables start to soften.

3. Stir in the corn kernels, black beans, and diced tomatoes with their juice. Mix well.

4. Add the vegetable broth, ground cumin, chili powder, paprika, dried oregano, salt, and pepper. Stir to combine all the flavors.

5. Bring the soup to a boil, then reduce the heat to low. Cover the pot and let the soup simmer gently for about 15-20 minutes, allowing the flavors to blend together and the vegetables to become tender.

6. Just before serving, squeeze the juice of one lime into the soup and stir.

7. Taste the soup and adjust the seasoning if needed. Add more chili powder for extra heat or more lime juice for tanginess.

8. Ladle the soup into bowls and garnish with chopped fresh cilantro.

9. Serve hot, with optional avocado slices on top for added creaminess and flavor.

CREAMY BROCCOLI SOUP

SERVINGS: 4 | CALORIES PER SERVING: 150KCAL | TOTAL COOKING TIME: 35 MINS

INGREDIENTS

2   cups broccoli florets, washed and chopped

1   small onion, chopped

2   cloves garlic, minced

2   cups low-sodium vegetable broth

1   cup unsweetened almond milk (or any milk of your choice)

1   medium potato, peeled and diced

1   tbsp olive oil

Salt and pepper to taste

Optonal toppings:
Fat-free Greek yogurt, chopped fresh herbs, grated cheese, toasted nuts

METHOD

1. Heat the olive oil in a large pot over medium heat. Add the chopped onion and garlic. Sauté for a few minutes until the onion becomes translucent.

2. Add the diced potato and chopped broccoli to the pot. Sauté for another 3-4 minutes, allowing the flavors to blend together.

3. Pour in the low-sodium vegetable broth. Bring the mixture to a boil, then reduce the heat to a simmer. Cover the pot and let it cook for about 15-20 minutes, or until the potato and broccoli are tender.

4. Once the vegetables are cooked, use an immersion blender to carefully blend the soup until smooth and creamy. Alternatively, you can transfer the mixture to a blender in batches and blend until smooth. Be cautious when blending hot liquids – allow the soup to cool slightly before blending and leave the blender lid slightly open to allow steam to escape.

5. Return the blended soup to the pot if you transferred it to a blender. Stir in the unsweetened almond milk (or your choice of milk). Add more milk if you prefer a thinner consistency.

6. Season the soup with salt and pepper to taste. Start with a small amount and adjust according to your preference.

7. Place the pot back on the stove and gently reheat the soup over a low heat, stirring occasionally to prevent sticking or burning. Be careful not to let the soup boil.

8. Once the soup is heated through, taste and adjust the seasoning if needed.

9. Serve the creamy broccoli soup hot. Ladle it into bowls and garnish with optional toppings such as a dollop of low-fat Greek yogurt, chopped fresh herbs (like parsley or chives), a sprinkle of grated cheese, or toasted nuts for added texture and flavor.

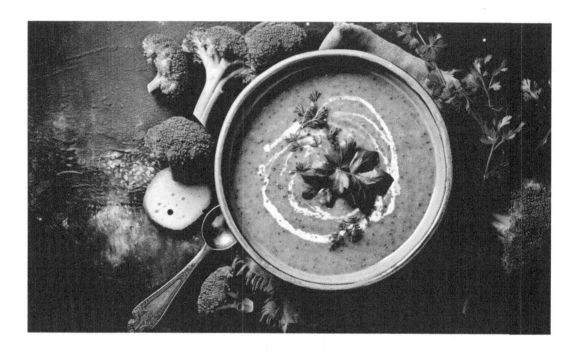

This recipe provides a nutritious and satisfying bowl of soup that's rich in fiber, vitamins, and minerals. It's a great way to enjoy the goodness of broccoli in a comforting and nourishing dish.

LEEK AND POTATO SOUP

SERVINGS: 4 | CALORIES PER SERVING: 150KCAL | TOTAL COOKING TIME: 35 MINS

INGREDIENTS

2   leeks, cleaned and thinly sliced (white and light green parts)

2   large potatoes, peeled and diced

1   onion, chopped

2   cloves garlic, minced

4   cups low-sodium vegetable broth

1   cup water

1   bay leaf

½   tsp dried thyme

½   tsp dried rosemary

½   tsp ground black pepper

¼   tsp salt (adjust to taste)

1   tbsp olive oil

½   cup unsweetened almond milk or low-fat milk (optional)

Fresh chives or parsley for garnish

When the weather is hot, leek and potato soup can quickly be transformed into chilled Vichyssoise. Simply cool the soup and chill in the refrigerator for at least two hours. Stir in a cup of fat free yogurt and serve in chilled bowls with a garnish of chopped parsley.

METHOD

1. Heat the olive oil in a large pot over medium heat. Add the chopped onion and cook for about 3-4 minutes until translucent.

2. Add the sliced leeks and minced garlic to the pot. Sauté for an additional 3-4 minutes until the leeks are softened.

3. Add the diced potatoes, dried thyme, dried rosemary, ground black pepper, and bay leaf to the pot. Stir everything together to coat the vegetables with the herbs and spices.

4. Pour in the vegetable broth and water. Bring the mixture to a boil, then reduce the heat to low, cover the pot, and let it simmer for about 20-25 minutes or until the potatoes are tender.

5. Remove the bay leaf from the soup and discard it.

6. Using an immersion blender, carefully blend the soup until smooth and creamy. If you don't have an immersion blender, you can blend the soup in batches using a regular blender. Be cautious when blending hot liquids.

7. If using, stir in the unsweetened almond milk or low-fat milk to add creaminess to the soup. This step is optional and can be omitted for a dairy-free or reduced calorie version.

8. Taste the soup and adjust the seasoning with salt and additional pepper if needed.

9. Serve hot, garnished with freshly chopped chives or parsley.

MEDITERRANEAN VEGETABLE SOUP

SERVINGS: 4 | CALORIES PER SERVING: 225KCAL | TOTAL COOKING TIME: 35 MINS

INGREDIENTS

- 2 tbsp olive oil
- 1 onion, diced
- 2 cloves garlic, minced
- 1 red bell pepper, diced
- 1 yellow bell pepper, diced
- 1 zucchini, diced
- 1 yellow squash, diced
- 1 carrot, peeled and diced
- 1 can (14 oz/400g) diced tomatoes, with juices
- 4 cups vegetable broth
- 1 tsp dried oregano
- 1 tsp dried thyme
- 1 tsp dried basil
- ½ tsp dried rosemary
- Salt and pepper to taste
- 1 cup cooked chickpeas (canned or cooked from dried)
- 2 cups fresh spinach or kale, chopped
- Juice of 1 lemon
- Fresh parsley, chopped, for garnish
- Crumbled feta cheese (optional), for serving

METHOD

1. Heat the olive oil in a large pot over medium heat. Add the diced onion and sauté for a few minutes until translucent.

2. Add the minced garlic and sauté for another 30 seconds until fragrant.

3. Add the diced red and yellow bell peppers, zucchini, yellow squash, and carrot to the pot. Sauté for about 5-7 minutes until the vegetables begin to soften.

4. Stir in the diced tomatoes (with their juice) and the vegetable broth.

5. Add the dried oregano, thyme, basil, rosemary, salt, and pepper to the pot. Stir well to combine.

6. Cover the pot and let the soup simmer for about 15-20 minutes, allowing the flavors to blend together.

7. Add the cooked chickpeas and chopped spinach or kale to the pot. Simmer for an additional 5-7 minutes until the greens are wilted.

8. Remove the pot from the heat and stir in the lemon juice. Taste and adjust the seasoning if needed.

9. Ladle the soup into serving bowls. Garnish with chopped fresh parsley and crumbled feta cheese, if desired.

This soup can be customized by adding other Mediterranean-inspired ingredients like olives, capers, or fresh herbs. It's not only delicious but also packed with nutritious vegetables, making it a perfect choice for a healthy and satisfying meal.

SPINACH AND WHITE BEAN SOUP

SERVINGS: 4 | CALORIES PER SERVING: 130KCAL | TOTAL COOKING TIME: 35 MINS

INGREDIENTS

1 tbsp olive oil

1 onion, chopped

2 cloves garlic, minced

2 carrots, peeled and diced

2 celery stalks, diced

1 tsp dried thyme

1 tsp dried rosemary

1 tsp ground cumin

4 cups low-sodium vegetable broth

2 (14 oz/400g) cans white beans, drained and rinsed

4 cups fresh baby spinach

Juice of 1 lemon

Salt and pepper to taste

Fresh parsley, chopped (for garnish)

METHOD

1. Heat the olive oil in a large pot over medium heat. Add the chopped onion and sauté until translucent, which should take around 3-4 minutes.

2. Add the minced garlic, diced carrots, and diced celery to the pot. Sauté for an additional 3-4 minutes, until the vegetables start to soften.

3. Stir in the dried thyme, dried rosemary, and ground cumin. Cook for another minute until the herbs become fragrant.

4. Pour in the low-sodium vegetable broth and bring the mixture to a simmer.

5. Add the drained and rinsed white beans to the pot. Stir well and let the soup simmer for about 15-20 minutes, allowing the flavors to blend together and the vegetables to become tender.

6. Using an immersion blender, carefully blend part of the soup to create a creamy base. You can blend as much or as little as you prefer, depending on the desired texture.

7. Stir in the fresh baby spinach and let it wilt into the soup.

8. Squeeze in the juice of one lemon to add brightness to the flavors. Season the soup with salt and pepper to taste.

9. Taste the soup and adjust the seasonings if needed. If the soup is too thick, you can add a little more vegetable broth to reach your desired consistency.

10. Serve the soup hot. Garnish with chopped fresh parsley before serving.

MOROCCAN HARIRA SOUP

SERVINGS: 6 | CALORIES PER SERVING: 140KCAL | TOTAL COOKING TIME: 55 MINS

INGREDIENTS

For the Soup:

1 cup dried chickpeas, soaked overnight and drained

1 tbsp olive oil

1 onion, finely chopped

2 cloves garlic, minced

2 carrots, peeled and diced

1 red bell pepper, diced

1 tsp ground cumin

1 tsp ground coriander

½ tsp ground turmeric

½ tsp ground cinnamon

¼ tsp ground ginger

¼ tsp ground paprika

¼ tsp ground black pepper

¼ tsp red pepper flakes (adjust to taste)

1 can (14 oz/400g) diced tomatoes

6 cups vegetable broth

½ cup green lentils

¼ cup chopped fresh parsley

¼ cup chopped fresh cilantro

Juice of 1 lemon

Salt to taste

For Garnish:

Chopped fresh parsley and cilantro

Lemon wedges (optional)

Hard-boiled eggs, chopped (optional)

Dates, chopped (optional)

METHOD

1. Heat the olive oil in a large pot over medium heat. Add the chopped onion and cook until it becomes translucent, for about 3-4 minutes.

2. Add the minced garlic and cook for another 1 minute, until fragrant.

3. Stir in the diced carrots and red bell pepper. Cook for about 5 minutes, until the vegetables start to soften.

4. Add the ground cumin, coriander, turmeric, cinnamon, ginger, paprika, black pepper, and red pepper flakes. Stir well to coat the vegetables with the spices.

5. Add the diced tomatoes (including their juice) to the pot and stir.

6. Pour in the vegetable broth and add the soaked and drained chickpeas and green lentils.

7. Bring the soup to a boil, then reduce the heat to low, cover the pot, and let the soup simmer for about 30-40 minutes, until the chickpeas and lentils are tender.

8. Once the chickpeas and lentils are cooked, stir in the chopped parsley and cilantro.

9. Just before serving, squeeze in the juice of one lemon and season the soup with salt to taste.

10. Ladle the soup into serving bowls. Garnish with additional chopped parsley and cilantro and serve with lemon wedges on the side.

11. If desired, you can also add chopped hard-boiled eggs and chopped dates to the soup for extra flavor and texture.

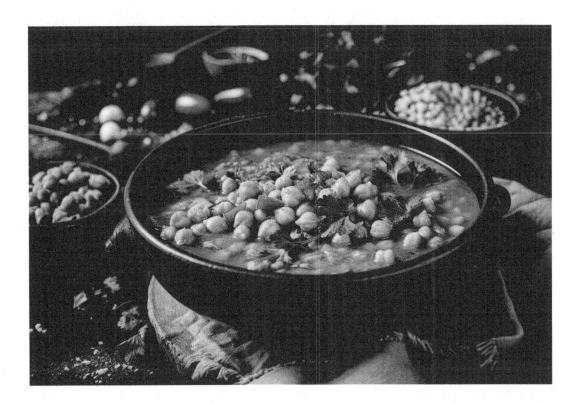

Harira soup is found in both Morocco and Algeria and differs as Algerian harira does not contain lentils. Moroccan Harira soup is traditionally eaten with dates and bread during Ramadan although it can be enjoyed all year around. It's a nourishing and comforting soup that's perfect for any occasion.

VEGAN

SOUP

RECIPES

CREAMY MUSHROOM SOUP

- -

SERVINGS: 4 | CALORIES PER SERVING: 175KCAL | TOTAL COOKING TIME: 35 MINS

INGREDIENTS

1 lb (450g) mushrooms, cleaned and sliced (use a mix of your favorite mushrooms)

1 medium onion, chopped

3 cloves garlic, minced

2 tbsp olive oil

3 cups vegetable broth

1 cup unsweetened almond milk or coconut milk

¼ cup raw cashews, soaked in hot water for about 20 minutes

2 tbsp nutritional yeast

1 tsp dried thyme

Salt and pepper to taste

Fresh parsley, chopped (for garnish)

METHOD

1. In a large pot, heat the olive oil over medium heat. Add the chopped onion and sauté for about 3-4 minutes until translucent.

2. Add the minced garlic and sliced mushrooms to the pot. Sauté for another 5-6 minutes until the mushrooms are tender and browned.

3. Pour in the vegetable broth and add the dried thyme. Bring the mixture to a simmer and let it cook for about 10 minutes, allowing the flavors to blend.

4. While the soup is simmering, drain the soaked cashews and add them to a blender along with the almond milk (or coconut milk) and nutritional yeast. Blend until smooth and creamy.

5. Carefully transfer the soup mixture to the blender with the cashew cream. Blend until the soup is smooth and creamy. You might need to do this in batches if your blender is not large enough to hold everything at once.

6. Return the blended soup to the pot and gently heat it over a low-medium heat. Season with salt and pepper to taste. If the soup is too thick, you can add a little more vegetable broth or almond milk to reach your desired consistency.

7. Once the soup is heated through, remove it from the heat.

8. Ladle the creamy mushroom soup into bowls and garnish with freshly chopped parsley.

9. Serve with your favorite crusty bread or a side salad for a complete and satisfying meal.

Enjoy this creamy soup that's dairy-free, vegan, and packed with flavor. The combination of sautéed mushrooms and cashew cream creates a rich and luxurious, velvety texture.

SPICY BLACK BEAN SOUP

SERVINGS: 4 | CALORIES PER SERVING: 220KCAL | TOTAL COOKING TIME: 35 MINS

INGREDIENTS

2   cans (14 ounces/400g each) black beans, drained and rinsed

1   tbsp olive oil

1   onion, diced

2-3 cloves garlic, minced

1   red bell pepper, diced

1   carrot, peeled and diced

1   tsp ground cumin

½   tsp smoked paprika

½   tsp chili powder (adjust to taste)

¼   tsp cayenne pepper (adjust to taste)

4   cups vegetable broth

1   can (14 oz/400g) diced tomatoes (with juice)

Juice of 1 lime

Salt and black pepper to taste

Fresh cilantro, chopped (for garnish)

Avocado slices (for garnish)

METHOD

1. In a large pot, heat the olive oil over medium heat. Add the diced onion and cook for about 3-4 minutes until it becomes translucent.

2. Add the minced garlic, diced red bell pepper and carrot, then sauté for another 5 minutes until the vegetables begin to soften.

3. Stir in the ground cumin, smoked paprika, chili powder, and cayenne pepper. Cook for an additional 1-2 minutes until the spices become fragrant.

4. Add the drained and rinsed black beans to the pot. Stir well to combine with the sautéed vegetables and spices.

5. Pour in the vegetable broth and diced tomatoes (with their juice). Bring the mixture to a boil, then reduce the heat to low and let it simmer for about 20-25 minutes to allow the flavors to blend.

6. Use an immersion blender to partially blend the soup, leaving some chunks of black beans and vegetables for texture. If you don't have an immersion blender, you can transfer a portion of the soup to a regular blender, blend, and then return it to the pot.

7. Stir in the lime juice and season the soup with salt and black pepper to taste. Adjust the spices if you want more heat.

8. Taste the soup and adjust the seasoning if needed. If you prefer a thinner consistency, you can add a little more vegetable broth.

9. Serve hot, garnished with chopped fresh cilantro and avocado slices.

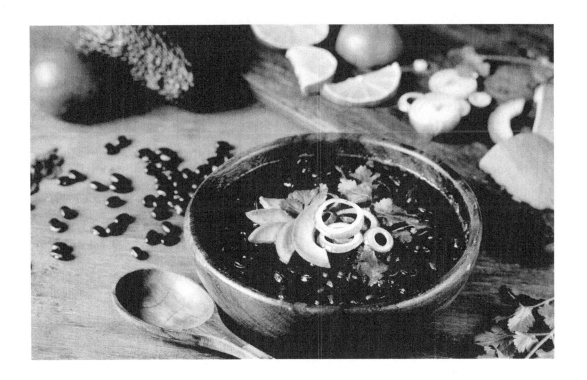

When appropriate, keep skins on vegetables for added fiber.

Add Greens: Throw in spinach, kale, or swiss chard for added vitamins.

Try hearty vegetables and legumes for a meat-free soup.

CURRIED CAULIFLOWER SOUP

SERVINGS: 4 | CALORIES PER SERVING: 235KCAL | TOTAL COOKING TIME: 35 MINS

INGREDIENTS

1 large cauliflower, chopped into florets

1 onion, chopped

2 cloves garlic, minced

1 tbsp curry powder

1 tsp ground cumin

½ tsp ground turmeric

½ tsp ground coriander

¼ tsp cayenne pepper (adjust to taste)

4 cups vegetable broth

1 can (14 oz/400g) coconut milk (full fat for creaminess)

1 tbsp olive oil

Salt and pepper to taste

Fresh cilantro or parsley, for garnish

Squeeze of fresh lemon juice (optional)

METHOD

1. In a large pot, heat the olive oil over medium heat. Add the chopped onion and sauté until translucent, about 3-4 minutes.

2. Add the minced garlic, curry powder, ground cumin, turmeric, ground coriander, and cayenne pepper. Sauté for another 1-2 minutes, stirring frequently, until the spices become fragrant.

3. Add the chopped cauliflower florets to the pot and stir well to coat them with the spice mixture. Cook for about 5 minutes, allowing the cauliflower to slightly soften.

4. Pour in the vegetable broth and bring the mixture to a boil. Reduce the heat to a simmer and cover the pot. Let the soup simmer for about 15-20 minutes, or until the cauliflower is tender.

5. Once the cauliflower is cooked, use an immersion blender to blend the soup until smooth and creamy. If you don't have an immersion blender, you can carefully transfer the soup in batches to a regular blender and blend until smooth.

6. Return the blended soup to the pot if needed. Stir in the coconut milk and heat the soup gently over low heat. Don't let it boil once the coconut milk is added to avoid curdling.

7. Season the soup with salt and pepper to taste. If desired, add a squeeze of fresh lemon juice for a touch of brightness.

8. Ladle the curried cauliflower soup into bowls and garnish with fresh cilantro or parsley leaves.

9. Serve warm with a slice of crusty bread or some wholegrain crackers.

CHICKPEA AND VEGETABLE SOUP

SERVINGS: 4 | CALORIES PER SERVING: 200KCAL | TOTAL COOKING TIME: 30 MINS

INGREDIENTS

1   tbsp olive oil

1   onion, chopped

2   cloves garlic, minced

2   carrots, peeled and diced

2   celery stalks, diced

1   red bell pepper, diced

1   zucchini, diced

1   tsp ground cumin

1   tsp ground coriander

½   tsp smoked paprika (optional)

¼   tsp turmeric

¼   tsp red pepper flakes (adjust to taste)

1   cup cooked chickpeas (canned or cooked from dried)

4   cups vegetable broth

1   can (14 oz/400g) diced tomatoes

1   bay leaf

2   cups chopped kale or spinach

Juice of 1 lemon

Salt and black pepper to taste

Fresh chopped parsley for garnish

METHOD

1. In a large pot, heat the olive oil over medium heat. Add the chopped onion and sauté until translucent, about 3-4 minutes.

2. Add the minced garlic and sauté for another 1 minute until fragrant.

3. Stir in the diced carrots, celery, red bell pepper, and zucchini. Cook for about 5 minutes, until the vegetables begin to soften.

4. Add the ground cumin, ground coriander, smoked paprika (if using), turmeric, and red pepper flakes. Stir to coat the vegetables with the spices and cook for another 1-2 minutes.

5. Pour in the cooked chickpeas, vegetable broth, diced tomatoes (with their juices), and bay leaf. Bring the soup to a simmer and let it cook for about 15-20 minutes, allowing the flavors to blend.

6. Add the chopped kale or spinach to the soup and let it cook for an additional 3-5 minutes, until the greens are wilted, then remove the bay leaf from the soup.

7. Stir in the lemon juice to add a refreshing tanginess. Season the soup with salt and black pepper to taste.

8. Ladle into serving bowls and garnish with chopped fresh parsley for a burst of color and freshness. Accompany the soup with crusty bread or your favorite wholegrain for a complete and satisfying vegan meal.

SWEET POTATO AND RED LENTIL SOUP

SERVINGS: 4 | CALORIES PER SERVING: 175KCAL | TOTAL COOKING TIME: 50 MINS

INGREDIENTS

1 tbsp olive oil

1 onion, chopped

2 cloves garlic, minced

1 tsp ground cumin

½ tsp ground turmeric

½ tsp ground ginger

¼ tsp ground cinnamon

1 large, sweet potato, peeled and diced

1 cup red lentils, rinsed and drained

4 cups vegetable broth

1 can (14 oz/400g) diced tomatoes (with juice)

Salt and pepper to taste

Juice of 1 lemon

Fresh cilantro or parsley, chopped (for garnish)

METHOD

1. In a large pot, heat the olive oil over medium heat. Add the chopped onion and sauté until translucent for around 4-5 minutes.

2. Add the minced garlic, ground cumin, turmeric, ginger, and cinnamon to the pot. Stir and cook for another 1-2 minutes until the spices become fragrant.

3. Add the diced sweet potato and red lentils to the pot. Stir to combine with the spices and onions.

4. Pour in the vegetable broth and diced tomatoes (including the juice). Stir well and bring the mixture to a boil.

5. Once the soup is boiling, reduce the heat to low, cover the pot, and let it simmer for about 20-25 minutes, or until the sweet potatoes and lentils are tender.

6. Using an immersion blender, carefully blend the soup until smooth and creamy. If you don't have an immersion blender, you can transfer the soup in batches to a regular blender and blend until smooth. Just be cautious when blending hot liquids.

7. Once the soup is blended, return it to the pot and heat it over low heat. If the soup is too thick, you can add more vegetable broth or water to achieve your desired consistency.

8. Season the soup with salt and pepper to taste. Squeeze in the juice of one lemon and stir to incorporate the flavors.

9. Serve hot, garnished with chopped fresh cilantro or parsley.

Enjoy this hearty and nutritious vegan soup that's packed with the goodness of sweet potatoes and red lentils. It's not only delicious but also full of fiber, vitamins, and plant-based protein.

VEGAN PHO

SERVINGS: 6 | CALORIES PER SERVING: 200KCAL | TOTAL COOKING TIME: 55 MINS

INGREDIENTS

For the Broth:

1 tbsp olive oil

8 cups vegetable broth

1 onion, sliced

3-4 garlic cloves, minced

2-inch piece of ginger, sliced

2 cinnamon sticks

3-4 star anise pods

4-5 cloves

1 tsp coriander seeds

1 tbsp soy sauce or tamari

1 tbsp coconut sugar
   or maple syrup
   Salt and pepper, to taste

For the Noodles and Toppings:

8 oz rice noodles
   (pho noodles)

1 cup sliced mushrooms
   (shiitake or oyster
   mushrooms work well)

1 cup bean sprouts

1 cup sliced bok choy
   or spinach

½ cup fresh herbs (cilantro,
   Thai basil, mint)

1 lime, cut into wedges
   Sriracha or chili
   sauce (optional)
   Hoisin sauce (optional)
   Sliced jalapenos (optional)

METHOD

1. In a large pot, heat the olive oil over medium heat. Add the chopped onion, minced garlic, and sliced ginger and sauté for about 3-4 minutes.

2. In a separate skillet, dry toast the cinnamon sticks, star anise, cloves, and coriander seeds for a couple of minutes until fragrant, before adding to the main pot.

3. Next, add the vegetable broth, soy sauce or tamari, and coconut sugar or maple syrup. Bring the mixture to a simmer and let it cook on low heat for about 20-30 minutes to infuse the flavors.

4. Strain the broth to remove the spices and aromatics. Return the strained broth to the pot and season with salt and pepper to taste. Keep the broth warm while you prepare the rest of the ingredients.

5. Cook the rice noodles according to the package instructions. Drain and rinse the noodles under cold water to prevent them from becoming too soft. Set aside.

6. In a separate pan, sauté the sliced mushrooms until they are tender and slightly browned. Set aside.

7. Prepare the toppings: Wash and chop the fresh herbs, slice the bok choy or spinach, and have the lime wedges, bean sprouts, and optional condiments ready.

8. To serve, divide the cooked rice noodles among serving bowls. Top the noodles with the sautéed mushrooms, sliced bok choy or spinach, and fresh herbs.

9. Ladle the hot broth over the noodles and toppings. The broth will slightly cook the vegetables.

10. Serve the vegan Pho bowls with lime wedges, bean sprouts, and optional condiments like Sriracha, hoisin sauce, and sliced jalapenos on the side.

11. Customize your Pho by adding the desired amount of condiments, herbs, and lime juice to suit your taste.

....

Balance acidity with a touch of sweetness, like a splash of apple cider vinegar.

....

....

Choose toppings like fat-free yogurt, fresh herbs, or a sprinkle of low-fat cheese.

....

....

A variety of colorful vegetables ensures diverse nutrients in your soup.

....

PEA AND MINT SOUP

· ·

SERVINGS: 4 | CALORIES PER SERVING: 185KCAL | TOTAL COOKING TIME: 35 MINS

INGREDIENTS

- 1 tbsp olive oil
- 1 small onion, chopped
- 2 cloves garlic, minced
- 4 cups frozen or fresh green peas
- 4 cups low sodium vegetable broth
- 1 medium potato, peeled and diced
- 1 little gem lettuce, washed and chopped
- ½ cup fresh mint leaves, plus extra for garnish
  Salt and pepper to taste
- ½ cup vegan coconut yogurt
  Lemon zest for garnish (optional)

METHOD

1. In a large pot, heat the olive oil over medium heat. Add the chopped onion and sauté for about 3-4 minutes until it becomes translucent. Add the minced garlic and continue to sauté for another minute until fragrant.

2. Add the green peas, lettuce, and diced potato to the pot. Stir for a minute to combine them with the onions and garlic.

3. Pour in the vegetable broth. Increase the heat to high and bring the mixture to a boil.

4. Once boiling, reduce the heat to low, cover the pot, and let it simmer for about 15-20 minutes, or until the peas and potatoes are tender.

5. Stir in the fresh mint leaves. Let the soup simmer for an additional 2-3 minutes to allow the mint flavor to infuse.

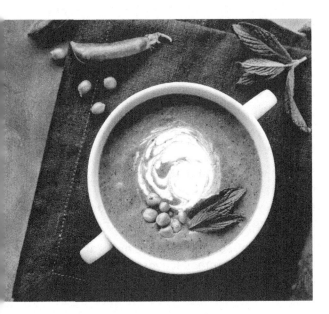

6. Using an immersion blender or a regular blender (in batches), carefully blend the soup until it's smooth and creamy.

7. Season the soup with salt and pepper to taste. Adjust the seasoning as needed.

8. Ladle into bowls. Swirl a spoonful of coconut yogurt (or other plant-based yogurt of your choice) into each bowl and garnish with extra fresh mint leaves and a sprinkle of lemon zest if desired.

WATERCRESS SOUP

SERVINGS: 4 | CALORIES PER SERVING: 125KCAL | TOTAL COOKING TIME: 30 MINS

INGREDIENTS

- 1   large bunch of fresh watercress (about 2 cups packed)
- 1   medium potato, peeled and diced
- 1   small onion, finely chopped
- 2   cloves garlic, minced
- 1   tbsp olive oil
- 4   cups low-sodium vegetable broth
- ½   cup vegan coconut yogurt
  Salt and pepper to taste
  Lemon wedges for garnish (optional)

METHOD

1. Wash the watercress thoroughly and remove any tough stems. Roughly chop the leaves and tender stems.

2. In a large pot, heat the olive oil over medium heat. Add the chopped onion and sauté for about 3-4 minutes until it becomes translucent. Stir in the minced garlic and cook for another 30 seconds until fragrant.

3. Add the diced potato and vegetable broth to the pot. Increase the heat to high and bring the mixture to a boil. Once boiling, reduce the heat to low, cover, and let it simmer for about 10-15 minutes or until the potato is tender.

4. Using an immersion blender or a regular blender (in batches), carefully purée the soup until smooth. If using a regular blender, allow the soup to cool slightly before blending and then reheat.

5. Return the soup to the pot (if using a regular blender) and place it over low heat. Stir in the chopped watercress and simmer for an additional 5 minutes. This will wilt the watercress and infuse the soup with its flavor.

6. Remove the pot from the heat. Stir in the coconut yogurt until well combined. This adds creaminess to the soup.

7. Season with salt and pepper to taste. Adjust the seasoning as needed. If desired, squeeze a lemon wedge over each serving for a refreshing zing.

8. Ladle the hot soup into bowls and garnish with extra watercress leaves or a dollop of yogurt, if desired. Serve immediately.

VEGAN MEXICAN TORTILLA SOUP

SERVINGS: 4 | CALORIES PER SERVING: 175KCAL | TOTAL COOKING TIME: 40 MINS

INGREDIENTS

For the Soup:

1 tbsp olive oil
1 onion, diced
2 cloves garlic, minced
1 red bell pepper, diced
1 jalapeño pepper, seeded and minced (adjust to your spice preference)
1 tsp ground cumin
1 tsp chili powder
½ tsp smoked paprika
1 can (14 oz/400g) diced tomatoes
4 cups vegetable broth
1 cup corn kernels (fresh, frozen, or canned)
1 can (14 oz/400g) black beans, drained and rinsed
Juice of 1 lime
Salt and pepper to taste

For Serving:

Tortilla chips, crushed
Avocado slices
Fresh cilantro leaves, chopped
Lime wedges
Fat-free plain coconut yogurt (optional)

METHOD

1. In a large pot, heat the olive oil over medium heat. Add the diced onion and cook for 2-3 minutes until it starts to soften.

2. Add the minced garlic, diced red bell pepper, and minced jalapeño pepper. Sauté for another 2-3 minutes until the peppers are slightly tender.

3. Stir in the ground cumin, chili powder, and smoked paprika. Cook for about 1 minute until the spices are fragrant.

4. Add the diced tomatoes with their juice and stir to combine. Let the mixture cook for a few minutes to allow the flavors to blend.

5. Pour in the vegetable broth and bring the soup to a simmer. Allow it to simmer for about 15-20 minutes to develop the flavors.

6. Add the corn kernels and black beans to the soup. Simmer for an additional 10 minutes.

7. Just before serving, squeeze in the juice of one lime and season the soup with salt and pepper to taste.

8. To serve, ladle the soup into bowls. Top each bowl with crushed tortilla chips, avocado slices, chopped cilantro, and a lime wedge. If desired, you can also add a dollop of dairy-free sour cream or coconut yogurt.

COCONUT CURRY SOUP

SERVINGS: 4 | CALORIES PER SERVING: 195KCAL | TOTAL COOKING TIME: 40 MINS

INGREDIENTS

For the Soup Base:

1   tbsp coconut oil
1   onion, diced
2   cloves garlic, minced
1   tbsp fresh ginger, minced
2   tbsp curry powder
1   tsp ground turmeric
1   tsp ground cumin
1   tsp ground coriander
1   can (14 oz/400g) diced tomatoes
1   can (14 oz/400g) coconut milk
4   cups vegetable broth
1   cup peeled and diced carrots
1   cup diced bell peppers
1   cup diced zucchini
     Salt and pepper to taste

For the Garnish:

Fresh cilantro, chopped
Lime wedges
Red pepper flakes (optional)
Sliced green onions

METHOD

1. In a large pot, heat the coconut oil over medium heat. Add the diced onion and cook until translucent, about 3-4 minutes.

2. Add the minced garlic and ginger, and sauté for another 1-2 minutes until fragrant.

3. Stir in the curry powder, ground turmeric, ground cumin, and ground coriander. Cook the spices for about 1 minute to release their flavors.

4. Add the diced tomatoes, coconut milk, and vegetable broth to the pot. Stir well to combine.

5. Add the diced carrots, bell peppers, and zucchini to the pot. Season with salt and pepper to taste. Bring the soup to a gentle boil, then reduce the heat to a simmer. Cover and let it simmer for about 15-20 minutes, or until the vegetables are tender.

6. Using an immersion blender or a regular blender (in batches if necessary), carefully blend the soup until smooth and creamy.

7. Taste and adjust the seasoning if needed. If you prefer a spicier soup, you can add red pepper flakes at this stage.

8. Once the soup is smooth and well-blended, ladle it into serving bowls.

9. Garnish each bowl with chopped fresh cilantro, a squeeze of lime juice, and sliced green onions and serve.

You can change this soup by adding other vegetables or protein sources like tofu or chickpeas.

MOROCCAN LENTIL SOUP

SERVINGS: 4 | CALORIES PER SERVING: 160KCAL | TOTAL COOKING TIME: 40 MINS

INGREDIENTS

1 cup red or brown lentils, rinsed and drained

1 large onion, finely chopped

3 cloves garlic, minced

2 carrots, peeled and diced

2 tomatoes, diced

1 red bell pepper, diced

1 tsp ground cumin

1 tsp ground coriander

½ tsp ground turmeric

½ tsp ground paprika

¼ tsp ground cinnamon

¼ tsp cayenne pepper (adjust to taste)

6 cups low-sodium vegetable broth

1 tbsp olive oil

Juice of 1 lemon

Salt and pepper to taste

Fresh cilantro or parsley for garnish

Lemon wedges for serving

METHOD

1. In a large pot, heat the olive oil over medium heat. Add the chopped onion and sauté for about 3-4 minutes, until translucent.

2. Add the minced garlic, ground cumin, ground coriander, ground turmeric, ground paprika, ground cinnamon, and cayenne pepper. Stir well and cook for another 1-2 minutes until fragrant.

3. Add the diced carrots, red bell pepper, and tomatoes to the pot. Cook for 5 minutes, stirring occasionally.

4. Add the rinsed lentils to the pot and pour in the vegetable broth. Stir to combine all the ingredients. Bring the mixture to a boil.

5. Once the soup is boiling, reduce the heat to low, cover the pot, and let it simmer for about 20-25 minutes or until the lentils are tender and cooked through.

6. Using an immersion blender or a regular blender, carefully blend the soup until it reaches your desired consistency. If using a regular blender, blend in batches and be cautious of the hot liquid.

7. Return the blended soup to the pot if using a regular blender. Stir in the lemon juice and season with salt and pepper to taste. Adjust the seasonings according to your preference.

8. Simmer the soup for an additional 5 minutes to allow the flavors to blend.

9. Serve the soup hot, garnished with fresh cilantro or parsley. You can also serve it with lemon wedges on the side for an extra citrusy kick.

ROASTED RED PEPPER SOUP

SERVINGS: 4 | CALORIES PER SERVING: 150KCAL | TOTAL COOKING TIME: 60 MINS

INGREDIENTS

3   red bell peppers, roasted, peeled, and seeds removed

1   medium onion, chopped

2   cloves garlic, minced

1   medium carrot, peeled and chopped

1   medium potato, peeled and chopped

3   cups vegetable broth

1   can (14 oz/400g) diced tomatoes (fire-roasted for extra flavor)

1   tsp smoked paprika

½   tsp ground cumin

¼   tsp cayenne pepper (adjust to taste)

1   tbsp olive oil

    Salt and pepper to taste

    Fresh chopped parsley (for garnish)

    Coconut yogurt (for topping, optional)

METHOD

1. Preheat the oven to 450°F (230°C).

2. Place the red bell peppers on a baking sheet and roast in the oven until the skins are charred and blistered, about 20-25 minutes.

3. Remove the peppers from the oven and immediately transfer them to a bowl. Cover the bowl with plastic wrap or a kitchen towel and let the peppers steam for about 15 minutes.

4. Once the peppers are cool enough to handle, peel off the charred skin, remove the seeds, and roughly chop the flesh. Set aside.

5. In a large pot, heat the olive oil over medium heat. Add the chopped onion and sauté until translucent, about 3-4 minutes.

6. Add the minced garlic, chopped carrot, and potato. Sauté for an additional 3-4 minutes.

7. Add the roasted red peppers, diced tomatoes (including their juices), smoked paprika, ground cumin, and cayenne pepper. Stir to combine.

8. Pour in the vegetable broth and bring the mixture to a boil. Reduce the heat to low, cover the pot, and let the soup simmer for about 15-20 minutes, or until the vegetables are tender.

9. Using an immersion blender or in batches in a countertop blender, carefully blend the soup until smooth and creamy. If using a countertop blender, return the blended soup to the pot.

10. Season the soup with salt and pepper to taste and reheat the soup if needed before serving.

11. Ladle the roasted red pepper soup into bowls, garnish with fresh chopped parsley and a drizzle of coconut yogurt if desired and serve!

CREAMY ASPARAGUS SOUP

SERVINGS: 4 | CALORIES PER SERVING: 150KCAL | TOTAL COOKING TIME: 40 MINS

INGREDIENTS

- 1 bunch of fresh asparagus, trimmed and chopped
- 1 medium onion, chopped
- 2 cloves garlic, minced
- 1 medium potato, peeled and diced into small cubes
- 4 cups vegetable broth
- 1 cup unsweetened almond milk (or any plant-based milk of your choice)
- 2 tbsp olive oil
- 1 tsp dried thyme
- Salt and pepper to taste
- Fresh lemon juice (optional, for garnish)
- Fresh chopped herbs (such as parsley or chives) for garnish

Asparagus is regarded as a spring superfood as it is packed with vitamins A, C, E, K and B6 as well as folate, copper, calcium, fiber, iron, and protein.

METHOD

1. In a large pot, heat the olive oil over medium heat. Add the chopped onion and sauté until translucent, about 3-4 minutes. Add the minced garlic and sauté for an additional 1-2 minutes until fragrant.

2. Add the diced potato, chopped asparagus, and dried thyme to the pot. Stir to combine and sauté for a couple of minutes.

3. Pour in the vegetable broth, ensuring that the vegetables are fully submerged. Bring the mixture to a boil, then reduce the heat to a simmer. Cover the pot and let the soup cook for about 15-20 minutes, or until the asparagus and potatoes are tender.

4. Once the vegetables are cooked, use an immersion blender to carefully blend the soup until smooth and creamy. If you don't have an immersion blender, you can transfer the soup in batches to a regular blender and blend until smooth. Just be sure to allow the soup to cool slightly before blending and vent the blender lid to prevent steam build-up.

5. Return the blended soup to the pot if needed and place it over low heat. Stir in the unsweetened almond milk (or other plant-based milk of your choice) to achieve the desired creamy consistency. Season with salt and pepper to taste. If the soup is too thick, you can add a little more vegetable broth or almond milk.

6. Taste the soup and adjust the seasonings as needed. If desired, squeeze in a little fresh lemon juice for a hint of brightness.

7. Serve hot, garnished with fresh chopped herbs of your choice. You can also drizzle a little olive oil or a swirl of plant-based yogurt on top for extra creaminess.

CREAMY ZUCCHINI SOUP

SERVINGS: 4 | CALORIES PER SERVING: 225KCAL | TOTAL COOKING TIME: 35 MINS

INGREDIENTS

1   tbsp olive oil

3   medium zucchinis, chopped

1   small onion, chopped

2   cloves garlic, minced

1   potato, peeled and chopped

4   cups vegetable broth

1   cup coconut milk (or
    any plant-based milk
    of your choice)

1   tsp dried thyme

    Salt and pepper to taste

    Fresh chopped herbs
    (such as parsley or
    chives) for garnish

METHOD

1. In a large pot, heat the olive oil over medium heat. Add the chopped onion and garlic and sauté until the onion becomes translucent.

2. Add the chopped zucchinis and potato to the pot. Cook for a few minutes, stirring occasionally.

3. Pour in the vegetable broth and add the dried thyme. Bring the mixture to a boil, then reduce the heat to a simmer. Cover the pot and let it cook for about 15-20 minutes, or until the zucchinis and potato are tender.

4. Remove the pot from the heat and allow it to cool slightly.

5. Using an immersion blender or a regular blender, carefully blend the soup until smooth and creamy. If using a regular blender, blend the soup in batches and be cautious of blending hot liquids.

6. Return the blended soup to the pot and place it back on the stove over a low heat.

7. Stir in the coconut milk (or other plant-based milk of your choice) to achieve the desired creaminess. You can add more or less milk depending on your preference.

8. Season the soup with salt and pepper to taste. Adjust the seasoning as needed.

9. Once the soup is heated through and seasoned, it's ready to be served.

10. Ladle the creamy soup into serving bowls. Garnish with fresh chopped herbs like parsley or chives and serve.

CARROT AND GINGER SOUP

SERVINGS: 4 | CALORIES PER SERVING: 250KCAL | TOTAL COOKING TIME: 40 MINS

INGREDIENTS

2 tbsp olive oil or coconut oil

6 large carrots, peeled and chopped

1 onion, chopped

2-3 cloves garlic, minced

1-inch piece of fresh ginger, peeled and minced

4 cups vegetable broth

1 can (14 oz/400g) coconut milk (full-fat for creamier soup)

1 tsp ground turmeric (optional, for color and flavor)

Salt and pepper to taste

Fresh cilantro or parsley, for garnish

METHOD

1. Heat the olive oil or coconut oil in a large pot over a medium heat. Add the chopped onion and sauté for a few minutes until translucent.

2. Add the minced garlic and ginger to the pot. Sauté for another minute until fragrant.

3. Add the chopped carrots to the pot and stir well to combine with the onion, garlic, and ginger.

4. Pour in the vegetable broth and bring the mixture to a boil. Reduce the heat to a simmer, cover the pot, and let it cook for about 20-25 minutes, or until the carrots are tender.

5. Once the carrots are cooked, remove the pot from the heat and use an immersion blender to carefully blend the soup until smooth and creamy. If you don't have an immersion blender, you can transfer the soup to a regular blender in batches, blend, and then return it to the pot.

6. Return the blended soup to the stovetop over a low heat. Stir in the coconut milk and ground turmeric (if using). Season with salt and pepper to taste. Allow the soup to warm through but avoid boiling it.

7. Taste the soup and adjust the seasonings if needed. If the soup is too thick, you can add a little more vegetable broth or water to achieve your desired consistency.

8. Once the soup is heated and seasoned to your liking, remove it from the heat.

9. Ladle into serving bowls. Garnish with fresh cilantro or parsley for a burst of flavor and color and serve.

This carrot and ginger soup is not only satisfying, but also rich in vitamins and antioxidants from the carrots and ginger.

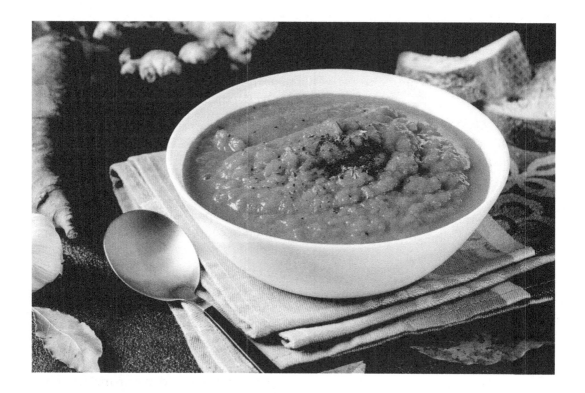

Well, that's it for the recipes, I'm sure you'll agree there's something in there for everyone, and some particularly tasty soups.

The last section of the book, I've dedicated to a range of information pages and cooking tips.

Depending on your level of expertise, you may already know a lot of what I cover, however, I'm confident there are some golden nuggets of advice that you will find useful, I know I certainly discovered a few new things when I was researching the book.

WHAT MAKES A HEALTHY DIET?

It's important to eat a wide range of healthy, wholesome foods in your diet each day, with a good balance of nutrients as well as vitamins, minerals, and water. The following nutritional percentages are recommended amounts based on a typical balanced diet for the average adult:

FATS

Fats provide essential energy to the body and are important for various bodily functions. Approximately 20-35% of your daily calorie intake should come from fats.

Here are some examples of fats -this is by no means an exhaustive list:

Saturated Fats: Butter, cheese, coconut oil, palm oil, animal fats (found in meat and dairy products)

Monounsaturated Fats: Olive oil, avocado, nuts (e.g., almonds, cashews, peanuts), seeds (e.g., pumpkin seeds, sesame seeds), canola oil

Polyunsaturated Fats: Fatty fish (e.g., salmon, mackerel, sardines), flaxseeds, chia seeds, sunflower oil, soybean oil

Trans Fats (Artificial Trans Fats, should be avoided as they are unhealthy): Processed foods (e.g., fried, and commercially baked goods), margarine, shortening

Omega-3 Fatty Acids (a type of polyunsaturated fat): Fatty fish (e.g., salmon, trout, herring), flaxseeds, chia seeds, walnuts

It's essential to include healthy fats in your diet, such as monounsaturated and polyunsaturated fats, which are found in many foods including avocados, nuts, seeds, olive oil, and fatty fish as they are nutritious and provide numerous health benefits. On the other hand, trans fats should be limited or even avoided, as they have been linked to various health issues and are often found in processed and fried foods.

As with any nutrient, it's important to consume fats in moderation as part of a balanced diet.

CARBOHYDRATES (CARBS)

Carbohydrates serve as an essential source of energy for the body. About 45-65% of your daily calorie intake should come from carbs. Choose complex carbohydrates found in whole grains, fruits, vegetables, and legumes over simple sugars found in sugary snacks, white bread, pastries, and beverages as these will take longer for your body to digest and keep you feeling fuller for longer.

Here are some examples of the most common carbohydrates:

Sugar: Including table sugar (sucrose), fructose (found in fruits), lactose (found in milk), and glucose (also known as dextrose, found in many foods).

Starch: Found in foods like potatoes, rice, corn, wheat, and other grains.

Fiber: Found in fruits, vegetables, whole grains, and legumes. Fiber is good for you as it is an indigestible carbohydrate that helps with digestion and promotes good gut health.

Bread and Baked Goods: Made from wheat or other grains, such as bread, bagels, muffins, and pastries.

Pasta: Made from wheat or other grains, such as spaghetti, macaroni, and lasagna.

Fruits: Such as apples, bananas, oranges, berries, and grapes.

Vegetables: Such as carrots, broccoli, sweet potatoes, and peas.

Legumes: Including beans, lentils, chickpeas, and peas.

Dairy Products: Such as milk, yogurt, and some types of cheese.

Sweets and Dessert: Including cookies, cakes, candies, and ice cream.

Try to include a variety of carbohydrates in your diet, focusing on complex carbohydrates (whole grains, fruits, vegetables, and legumes) for more sustained energy and better nutritional value. Simple carbohydrates (sugars and processed foods like white bread) should be consumed in moderation, as they can lead to rapid spikes and drops in blood sugar levels.

PROTEINS

Roughly 10-35% of your daily calorie intake should come from protein food groups. Always opt for lean types of protein like poultry, fish, beans, lentils, tofu, and low-fat dairy.

Here are some examples of foods that are sources of proteins:

MEAT: Beef, chicken, pork, lamb, and other types of meat are rich sources of protein.

POULTRY: Chicken and turkey are excellent sources of lean protein.

FISH: Salmon, tuna, cod, trout, and other types of fish are high in protein and also provide healthy omega-3 fatty acids.

EGGS: Eggs are a complete protein source and can be prepared in various ways.

DAIRY PRODUCTS: Milk, yogurt, cheese, and other dairy products are good sources of protein, especially cottage cheese and Greek yogurt -low fat options are best.

LEGUMES: Beans, lentils, chickpeas, and peas are plant-based sources of protein.

NUTS AND SEEDS: Almonds, peanuts, chia seeds, sunflower seeds, and pumpkin seeds are rich in protein and healthy fats.

TOFU AND TEMPEH: These soy-based products are popular among vegetarians and vegans for their protein content.

QUINOA: A pseudo-grain that is a complete protein source and a staple in many international diets.

EDAMAME: Young, green soybeans that are a popular protein-rich snack or addition to salads.

GREEK YOGURT: High in protein and calcium, Greek yogurt is a popular choice for breakfast or snacks.

COTTAGE CHEESE: A dairy product rich in protein, commonly eaten as a snack or added to salads.

SEITAN: Made from wheat gluten, seitan is a high-protein meat substitute used in many vegetarian dishes.

PROTEIN BARS: Many protein bars are designed to provide a convenient source of protein on the go, however many are also full of sugars and artificial sweeteners, so be wary of this.

Remember that proteins are essential for various bodily functions, including muscle repair and growth, immune system support, and enzyme production. You should include a variety of protein sources in your diet to ensure you're getting all the essential amino acids and nutrients your body needs.

ESSENTIAL KITCHEN EQUIPMENT AND TOOLS

Here are just some of the essential kitchen tools and equipment that can make cooking and baking more efficient and enjoyable. Having a well-equipped kitchen or at least a range of good basic tools can enhance your overall cooking experience and make it easier to try out new recipes.

Cutting Board: A good quality cutting board is essential for chopping, slicing, and dicing ingredients safely and efficiently.

Chef's Knife: A sharp and versatile chef's knife is a must-have for various cooking tasks, including cutting vegetables, meat, and herbs.

Measuring Cups and Spoons: Accurate measurements are crucial for successful cooking and baking. Invest in a set of measuring cups and spoons for precise ingredient quantities. Always use the same cup or spoon measures.

Mixing Bowls: Various sizes of mixing bowls are handy for mixing, whisking, and combining ingredients.

Baking Sheet: Baking sheets are versatile and used for baking cookies, roasting vegetables, and more.

Saucepan and Skillet: These are essential for stovetop cooking, such as making sauces, soups, and sautéing.

Pot with Lid: A pot with a lid is essential for boiling water, cooking grains, and preparing soups and stews.

Wooden Spoon: A wooden spoon is gentle on cookware and is ideal for stirring and mixing ingredients.

Whisk: Whisks are perfect for incorporating air into mixtures and beating eggs.

Spatula: A spatula is useful for flipping and turning food items in pans without damaging them.

Colander: A colander is essential for draining pasta, washing vegetables, and straining liquids.

Blender or Food Processor: A blender or food processor is handy for making smoothies, sauces, and purees.

Oven Mitts: Oven mitts are necessary for handling hot dishes and baking trays safely.

Thermometer: A cooking thermometer is useful for checking the internal temperature of meats and baked goods.

Grater: A grater is essential for grating (shredding) cheese, zesting citrus, and grating vegetables.

Rolling Pin: A rolling pin is needed for rolling out dough for baked goods and pastry.

Cooking Parchment: Cooking parchment paper is great for lining baking sheets and really prevents sticking.

Can Opener: For opening canned ingredients easily.

Kitchen Timer: A timer helps in keeping track of cooking and baking times.

Vegetable Peeler: Handy for peeling vegetables and fruits.

BASIC FOOD PREPARATION TIPS

Use a sharp knife: A sharp knife makes cutting easier and safer, reducing the risk of accidents.

Practice the claw grip: Curl your fingers under while holding the food you're chopping to protect them while prepping food.

Learn basic knife cuts: Master techniques like chopping, dicing, slicing, and julienne (matchsticks) for efficient prep work.

Use a mandolin slicer: For thin and uniform slices, a mandolin slicer is a handy tool.

Invest in a good pair of kitchen shears: They are useful for cutting herbs, trimming meats, and opening packaging.

Crush garlic with the flat side of a knife: Press down on a garlic clove with the flat side of a knife to easily remove the skin.

Cut onions properly: Slice off the stem end, cut in half, peel, and then make horizontal cuts before dicing.

Trim vegetables efficiently: Trim the ends of vegetables in a batch to save time.

Use a food processor: A food processor can quickly chop, grate, and slice ingredients and is worth using if you have a lot of things to prepare.

Prep in advance: Spend some time at the weekend prepping ingredients for the week ahead or batch cooking.

FOOD PREP TIME-SAVING TIPS

Buy pre-cut and pre-washed produce: Convenience products can save time during busy weekdays.

Use frozen fruits and vegetables: They are already prepared and ready for use, cutting down on prep time and also may actually contain more vitamins and minerals than the fresh version.

Buy pre-marinated meats if you can: Pre-marinated meats add flavor without requiring extra prep work.

Plan simple meals: Choose recipes with minimal prep work for busy days.

Cook once, eat twice: Make larger batches of ingredients and repurpose them into different meals.

Keep your kitchen organized: A well-organized kitchen saves time searching for tools and ingredients.

HOW TO STORE FRESH PRODUCE

o Store herbs with stems in water: Place fresh herbs like cilantro and parsley in a glass of water and cover them with a plastic bag for extended freshness.

o Keep onions and potatoes separate: Onions release gases that can cause potatoes to spoil faster, so store them separately.

o Store tomatoes at room temperature: Tomatoes lose flavor and texture when refrigerated.

o Keep berries dry: Store berries in a single layer on a paper towel in a breathable container to prevent the growth of mold.

o Store leafy greens with a damp paper towel: Keep greens fresh longer by storing them in a plastic bag with a slightly damp paper towel.

o Store citrus fruits in the fridge: Citrus fruits stay fresher when refrigerated.

o Wrap celery in foil: Wrapping celery in foil helps retain its crispness.

o Store mushrooms in a paper bag: Avoid plastic bags, which can trap moisture and cause mushrooms to spoil.

Use airtight containers: Store prepped ingredients in airtight containers to maintain freshness and prevent odors from spreading.

BEGINNERS GUIDE TO COOKING TECHNIQUES

Cooking techniques refer to methods used to prepare food. Each technique has its unique purpose and effect on the various ingredients, resulting in different textures, flavors, and appearances. Here are some common cooking techniques:

BOILING: Involves cooking food in boiling water or liquid. It is commonly used for pasta, vegetables, and eggs. Boiling helps to cook food quickly and can soften vegetables while preserving their nutrients.

SIMMERING: Similar to boiling, but the liquid is kept at a lower temperature, just below boiling point so the water very gently bubbles. It is ideal for cooking stews, soups, and braising meats, as the slower cooking allows flavors to blend together.

STEAMING: Cooking food with steam, usually done in a steamer or with a covered pot. Steaming retains more of the food's nutrients and natural flavors, making it a healthy cooking method for vegetables, fish, and dumplings.

FRYING: Involves cooking food in hot oil or fat. There are two main types of frying:

- **Deep Frying:** Submerging food completely in hot oil, resulting in a crispy texture. Common foods include French fries, fried chicken, and donuts.
- **Shallow Frying:** Cooking food in a small amount of oil, just enough to cover the bottom of the pan. It is often used for sautéing vegetables, omelets, or cooking pancakes.

SAUTÉING: Quickly cooking food in a small amount of oil or butter over high heat. It is used for vegetables, meat, or seafood and creates a flavorful, lightly browned exterior.

GRILLING: Cooking food directly over an open flame or heat source. Grilling adds a smoky flavor and attractive grill marks to meats, vegetables, and even fruits.

ROASTING: Cooking food in the oven at a higher temperature, typically used for larger cuts of meat, whole poultry, and vegetables. Roasting brings out rich flavors and caramelization.

BAKING: Cooking food by surrounding it with dry, hot air in an oven. Baking is commonly used for cakes, cookies, bread, and casseroles.

BROILING/GRILLING: Cooking food under direct heat, usually from an overhead heat source in the oven. Broiling is used to quickly cook or brown the top of dishes like fish fillets or gratins.

BRAISING: Combining both dry-heat and moist-heat cooking methods. It involves searing food in a pan, then simmering it in liquid at a low temperature. Braising is used for tough cuts of meat, making them tender and flavorful.

POACHING: Cooking food gently in liquid below its boiling point. Poaching is often used for delicate items like eggs, fish, and fruits.

MARINATING: Soaking food in a seasoned liquid, known as a marinade, to add flavor and tenderize the ingredients. Commonly used for meats and vegetables before grilling or roasting.

FOOD SUBSTITUTES FOR COMMON ALLERGIES OR DIETARY PREFERENCES

It's not always possible to follow a recipe exactly. There may be many reasons why you need to switch out an ingredient or two such as allergies, taste preferences, to save money or to simply use the ingredients you already have. Here is a selection of food substitutes that you can use:

Egg Substitutes:
- **For binding:** Applesauce, mashed banana, or pumpkin puree.
- **For leavening:** Baking powder or baking soda mixed with vinegar or lemon juice.
- **For moisture:** Yogurt, buttermilk, or non-dairy milk like almond, oat, or soy milk.

Milk Substitutes:
- **Cow's milk:** Almond milk, soy milk, oat milk, coconut milk, rice milk, or hemp milk.
- **Buttermilk:** Add 1 tablespoon of vinegar or lemon juice to a cup of non-dairy milk and let it sit for 5 minutes.

Wheat Flour Substitutes:
- **Gluten-free flours:** Almond flour, coconut flour, rice flour, quinoa flour, buckwheat flour, potato flour or chickpea flour.

Nut Allergies:
- **Nut butters:** Sunflower seed butter, pumpkin seed butter, or soy nut butter.
- **Nut toppings:** Toasted seeds, shredded coconut, or crushed pretzels.

Dairy Butter Substitutes:
- Coconut oil, vegan butter, margarine, or vegetable shortening.

Soy Substitutes:
- **Tofu:** Use chickpea tofu, tempeh, or lentils for a similar texture and protein content.
- **Soy sauce:** Tamari (gluten-free), coconut aminos, or liquid aminos.

Fish and Shellfish Substitutes:
- **Plant-based alternatives:** Tofu, tempeh, jackfruit, or heart of palm can mimic seafood textures.

- **Seaweed:** Nori or dulse can add a fishy flavor to dishes.

Meat Substitutes:
- **Beans and legumes:** Lentils, chickpeas, black beans, or kidney beans can replace meat in various dishes.
- **Plant-based meat substitutes:** Quorn, mycoprotein, or other commercially available meat alternatives.

Gluten Substitutes (for baking):
- Xanthan gum or guar gum can help provide structure to gluten-free baked goods.
- Arrowroot starch, tapioca starch, or corn starch can help thicken sauces and gravies.

Sugar Substitutes:
- **Honey:** Maple syrup, agave nectar, or date syrup.
- **Granulated sugar:** Coconut sugar, stevia, or erythritol for low-calorie options.

TROUBLESHOOTING TIPS FOR COMMON COOKING CHALLENGES

Every chef or accomplished cook has had their fair share of cooking disasters, it's just a natural part of the process. One moments lapse in concentration, or a misread recipe, you name it and anyone who cooks regularly will have experienced it. Here's my list of top tips for winning in the kitchen.

Overcooking:

Use a timer: Set a timer when cooking to avoid overcooking. Keep an eye on the cooking process and check the food regularly to prevent it from becoming overdone.

Lower heat: Reduce the heat if you notice the food cooking too quickly. Lowering the temperature allows for more even cooking and prevents burning.

Use a meat thermometer: For meats, use a thermometer to check the internal temperature. This way, you can ensure that the meat is cooked to the desired level without overcooking it.

Undercooking:

Increase cooking time: If you find that the food is undercooked, extend the cooking time. Keep in mind that different ovens and stovetops may vary in temperature, so adjust accordingly.

Slice or dice smaller: For larger or thicker pieces of food, consider slicing or dicing them smaller. This can help the food cook more evenly and thoroughly.

Precook tough ingredients: If certain ingredients take longer to cook, consider pre-cooking or blanching them before adding them to the dish.

Poor taste (Adjusting Seasoning):

Taste and adjust: Regularly taste your food as you cook. If you find that the dish lacks flavor, start by adding small amounts of salt and other seasonings, tasting after each addition until it reaches the desired taste.

Balancing flavors: If a dish is too salty, add a bit of acidity (like lemon juice or vinegar) or sweetness (like sugar or honey) to balance the flavors. For dishes that are too spicy, consider adding dairy, like yogurt or sour cream, to mellow the heat.

Use fresh herbs and spices: Fresh herbs and spices have more potent flavors than dried ones. Consider using fresh ingredients to enhance the dish's taste.

Incorporate layers of flavor: Building layers of flavor can improve the taste of a dish. Start by sautéing aromatics like onions and garlic, then add herbs, spices, and other seasonings as you go.

Don't rush: Sometimes, allowing the dish to simmer or rest can help the flavors blend together and develop over time.

Be cautious with salt: Be mindful of the amount of salt you add, as it is easier to add more salt than to remove it. If you accidentally add too much salt, you can try diluting it by adding more of the other ingredients or using water or broth instead.

Remember, cooking is a skill, and adjustments might be necessary to achieve the desired results. Don't be afraid to experiment and make changes to recipes to suit your taste preferences.

HOW TO MAKE YOUR FOOD LOOK AND TASTE BETTER

Enhancing the visual appeal of dishes through garnishing and plating can elevate the overall look and feel of your food, from dull and tasteless, to exciting and full of flavor. Here are some garnishing ideas and tips to help you create visually better-looking plates:

o **USE FRESH HERBS:** Sprinkle or place fresh herbs like basil, parsley, cilantro, or chives on top of the dish. They add a pop of color and a touch of freshness to the presentation.

o **EDIBLE FLOWERS:** Edible flowers like nasturtiums, pansies, or violets can add a beautiful and delicate touch to salads, desserts, or savory dishes.

o **CITRUS ZEST:** Grate or sprinkle citrus zest (lemon, lime, or orange) over the dish to add vibrant color and a burst of flavor.

o **SAUCE DRIZZLE:** Use a spoon or squeeze bottle to drizzle a colorful sauce or coulis on the plate. It adds visual interest and complements the flavors of the meal.

o **MICROGREENS:** These tiny, young greens are packed with flavor and make great garnishes. Using microgreens like radish, arugula, or pea shoots adds a sophisticated touch.

o **PLAY WITH TEXTURES:** Incorporate different textures on the plate to make it visually appealing. Crispy elements, creamy sauces, and crunchy toppings can all add dimension to the dish.

o **PLATE IN ODD NUMBERS:** Placing items in odd numbers (e.g., three cherry tomatoes or five asparagus spears) can create a more aesthetically pleasing arrangement.

o **BALANCE COLORS:** Consider the color composition of the plate. A mix of vibrant colors can make the dish look more enticing. However, avoid overcrowding the plate with too many colors.

- o **USE DIFFERENT PLATING TOOLS:** Explore various plating tools like tweezers, ring molds, or paintbrushes to achieve more precise and artistic arrangements.

- o **NEGATIVE SPACE:** Leave some empty or negative space on the plate to allow the main elements to stand out. It provides a cleaner and more focused presentation.

- o **LAYERING:** Create depth and visual interest by layering different components of the dish. For example, place a stack of vegetables or proteins over a bed of grains or puree.

- o **GARNISH WITH NUTS AND SEEDS:** Sprinkle toasted nuts or seeds like sesame, sunflower, or pumpkin seeds over the dish for added texture and flavor.

- o **USE COLORFUL PLATES:** Select plates that complement the colors of the dish. White plates often provide an excellent canvas for showcasing the food's vibrancy.

- o **KEEP IT SIMPLE:** While garnishing is essential, remember not to overwhelm the dish with too many elements. Sometimes, a simple, elegant garnish can be more impactful.

BE PLAYFUL: Have fun and get creative with your garnishing. Playful and artistic touches can make the dish more visually appealing.

Remember, with presentation there are no strict rules. So why try experimenting to find your own unique style and create visually stunning dishes that leave a lasting impression on your guests.

STORAGE AND REHEATING TIPS

Proper storage and reheating of leftovers are crucial for ensuring food safety and preserving the flavor and texture of the food. Here are some instructions to follow:

Storage

Refrigerate Promptly: After cooking, cool the leftovers as quickly as possible. Divide large portions into smaller containers to speed up cooling. Always aim to refrigerate the leftovers within two hours of cooking.

Proper Containers: Use airtight containers or resealable plastic bags for storage. Ensure the containers are clean and food safe.

Label and Date: Always label the containers with the name of the food and the date it was stored. This will help you keep track of how long the leftovers have been in the fridge.

Storage Temperature: Set your refrigerator to 40°F (4°C) or below to maintain the freshness of the leftovers. Avoid overloading the refrigerator, as it can affect the cooling efficiency.

Keep Raw and Cooked Foods Separate: Store raw and cooked foods separately to prevent cross-contamination.

Reheating

Reheat Thoroughly: When reheating leftovers, make sure they reach an internal temperature of 165°F (74°C) throughout. Use a food thermometer to check the temperature.

Avoid Reheating Multiple Times: Reheat leftovers only once. Repeated reheating can lead to bacterial growth and affect the taste and texture of the food.

Use Microwaves Safely: If using a microwave, stir the food during reheating to ensure even heating. Cover the container to trap steam and prevent drying out.

Oven Reheating: For larger portions, reheating in the oven is ideal. Cover the dish with foil to retain moisture and prevent burning.

Stovetop Reheating: Reheat soups, stews, and sautéed dishes on the stovetop over medium heat. Stir occasionally to prevent sticking.

Gravy and Sauces: Reheat gravies and sauces on the stovetop, adding a little water or broth to maintain the desired consistency.

Avoid Overcooking: Reheat just until the food is hot throughout. Overcooking can lead to loss of moisture and affect the taste.

Check for Spoilage: If leftovers have a strange odor, strange appearance, or an unusual texture, discard them immediately. It's better to be safe than sorry.

General Tips:

Use Leftovers Within 3-4 Days: Consume leftovers within three to four days to ensure freshness and safety. If you can't eat them in time, consider storing in a refrigerator or freezing them for longer storage.

Freezing Leftovers: If you have large amounts of leftovers that weren't cooked from frozen, consider freezing them in individual portions. When required, simply thaw them in the refrigerator and then reheat as needed.

Defrost Properly: If reheating frozen leftovers, thaw them in the refrigerator overnight. Avoid thawing at room temperature to prevent bacterial growth.

By following these storage and reheating instructions, you can enjoy safe and delicious leftovers while minimizing food waste and maintaining food quality. Always prioritize food safety to protect yourself and your family from foodborne illnesses.

MEASUREMENT CONVERSION CHARTS

CUPS	OUNCES (oz)	GRAMS (g)
¼ cup	0.8 oz	22.5g
½ cup	1.5 oz	45g
1 cup	3 oz	85g
1 ½ cups	4.5 oz	135g
2 cups	6.5 oz	180g
3 cups	9.5 oz	270g
OUNCES (oz)	**GRAMS (g) Approx.**	**GRAMS (g) Exact**
1 oz	25g	28.3g
2 oz	50g	56.6g
3 oz	75g	84.9g
4 oz	100g	113.2g
5 oz	125g	141.5g
6 oz	150g	169.8g
7 oz	175g	198.1g
8 oz	200g	227.0g

Serving Size	OUNCES (oz)
¼ tsp	1.25ml
½ tsp	2.5ml
1 tsp	5 ml
1 tbsp	15 ml
¼ cup	2 fluid ozs
½ cup	4 fluid ozs
1 cup	8 fluid ozs
2 cups	13 fluid ozs
3 cups	26 fluid ozs

tsp = teaspoon, tbsp = tablespoon, ml = milliliters

ABOUT THE AUTHOR

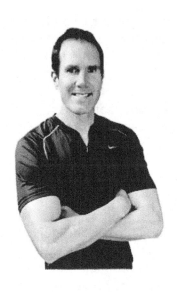

Please allow me to introduce myself. My name is Jago Holmes, and I am the author and creator of *"Healthy Soups For Healthy Living,"* a book which showcases a wide range of healthy, nutritious soups from all around the world. I am also the owner and principal trainer here at New Image Personal Training in Halifax, England. We regularly work with over 100 clients every week in our exclusive 1:1 studio.

I am a fully qualified and experienced fitness trainer and weight loss expert. My personal training company has been in operation for more than 20 years now and we consistently get great results with our clients, and so I'd like to share my knowledge and success with you now.

I've written hundreds of magazine articles as well as countless blogs and numerous website posts and have created a range of digital e-books and weight loss packages. I regularly presented fat loss seminars as well as running my acclaimed *8 Week Weight Loss Challenge.*

I studied at the University of Leeds, completing my training with the YMCA in 2000. After three years, I attained the YMCA Personal Trainer Award - one of the highest and most respected qualifications in the UK for Personal Trainers.

I have a lifetime love and passion for all things related to health and fitness and this helps me to think 'outside the box' in search of solutions to many of my client's most challenging situations.

Lack of time, medical conditions, food intolerances, lack of motivation, unusual working patterns, limited budgets… you name it, and the chances are I have worked with a client who has had that exact same problem.

As a result of this, I have created a range of books that address many of these needs and more.

It's amazing how one piece of knowledge, clever tip or trick can literally change someone's life around -instantly transforming the way they think about their own circumstances. I like to look for answers from outside the usual places that most people search.

What I've tried to do with my books is to write in an easy-to-understand style that gives the answers to questions that people need without being blinded by science.

My books are not meant for academics or boffins, they're meant to be read and understood by everyday people. I try to add unusual or little-known techniques into what I write that people can use because they have been proven to be effective in all manner of ways.

Often, we look to the most obvious answers for losing weight... eating less and exercising more. Whilst this is certainly the answer in many cases, sometimes there are other issues present and things that can be done differently.

In my writing, this is what I'm looking for -ways of doing things differently and more effectively that can make a real difference to people's lives.

I hope you enjoy reading my book and put into action the steps, techniques, tips, and advice that you learn. If you like what you've read and think others would also benefit, then please leave your positive comments for others to learn about your experience as it makes the Amazon marketplace a much more honest and enjoyable place for people to shop and buy books.

If you can think of any ways that you feel this book could be improved, please send an email to me – jago@jagoholmes.com and I'll try to add your suggestions.

To your health and fitness,

Jago Holmes CPT
Personal Trainer and Weight Loss Expert

WALKING FOR WEIGHT LOSS

A fantastic weight loss walking program with four unique and HIGHLY effective walking techniques -The easiest and most effective way to blast through stubborn fat stores at the fastest rate possible.

This book will help anyone lose weight. *It's an effective alternative for those who don't want to use a gym/fitness class or hate the idea of going running.* Go here to find out more about a unique fat burning system you can start today:

https://www.amazon.com/dp/B0C53WR3G4

THE APPLE CIDER VINEGAR WEIGHT LOSS REVOLUTION

In this ground-breaking book, you can discover the secrets behind apple cider vinegar's ability to accelerate fat burning, boost metabolism, curb cravings, and enhance digestion.

Backed by scientific research and centuries of traditional use, this book provides a step-by-step roadmap to help you harness the full potential of apple cider vinegar for your own body transformation and weight loss success.

Go here to discover more about the amazing benefits of ACV:

https://www.amazon.com/dp/B0CFL6JKYM

THE COCONUT FLOUR COOKBOOK

Indulge in your favorite comfort foods guilt-free! With "The Coconut Flour Cookbook," you can recreate classic dishes like pancakes, muffins, bread, and cookies, without compromising on taste or nutrition. Embrace a healthier lifestyle while enjoying the flavors you love.

Unlock the culinary wonders of coconut flour and revolutionize your cooking today! Go here to grab your copy of "The Coconut Flour Cookbook":

https://www.amazon.com/dp/B00CSTZ94I

Made in United States
North Haven, CT
31 August 2024

56777999R00109